Forensic Radiology

FORENSIC RADIOLOGY

K. T. EVANS

M.B., Ch.B., F.R.C.P., D.M.R.D., F.R.C.R.,
F.F.R. (R.C.S.I.)
Professor of Diagnostic Radiology
Welsh National School of Medicine
Cardiff

B. KNIGHT

M.D., B.Ch., F.R.C.Path., D.M.J., Barrister at Law
Professor of Forensic Pathology
Welsh National School of Medicine
Cardiff
Home Office Pathologist

With contributions from

D. K. WHITTAKER

B.D.S., Ph.D., F.D.S., R.C.S.
Senior Lecturer in Oral Biology
Welsh National School of Medicine
Cardiff
Home Office Forensic Odontologist

Blackwell Scientific Publications

Oxford London Edinburgh
Boston Melbourne

© 1981 by
Blackwell Scientific Publications
Editorial offices:
Osney Mead, Oxford, OX2 0EL
8 John Street, London, WC1N 2ES
9 Forrest Road, Edinburgh, EH1 2QH
52 Beacon Street, Boston
   Massachusetts 02108, USA
214 Berkeley Street, Carlton
   Victoria 3053, Australia

First published 1981

Printed in Great Britain
at the Alden Press, Oxford
and bound at Kemp Hall Bindery

Distributors

USA
   Blackwell Mosby Book Distributors
   11830 Westline Industrial Drive
   St Louis, Missouri 63141

Canada
   Blackwell Mosby Book Distributors
   120 Melford Drive, Scarborough
   Ontario, M1B 2X4

Australia
   Blackwell Scientific Book Distributors
   214 Berkeley Street, Carlton
   Victoria 3053

British Library
Cataloguing in Publication Data
Evans, K.T.
   Forensic radiology.
   1. Forensic radiography
   I. Title   II. Knight, B.
   III. Whittaker, D.K.
   616.07'57   RA1058.5

   ISBN 0 632 00587 4

Contents

Preface

Contact between radiology and the law occurs much more frequently than might be expected—and it occurs over a wide spectrum of situations. These fall into two main categories—those where radiological methods are deliberately employed to investigate some forensic problem and those where the practice of radiology itself gives rise to some medico-legal consequences.

The first group is exemplified by the increasing assistance that the forensic pathologist obtains from his radiological colleagues, most often in special investigations related to post-mortem examination. The identification of skeletal and dental material, the location of missiles and foreign bodies and the detection of bone injuries are prime examples of this assistance.

A much wider and more diffuse field where radiology has an interface with jurisprudence and medical ethics, occurs when the professional activities and conduct of the radiologist becomes the subject of legal notice. This has become increasingly important in recent years, due to the rapid advances in radiological techniques and the increasing complexity and potential hazard of some diagnostic procedures. Matters such as informed consent and responsibility for real or alleged negligence are in the forefront of this category.

This book is a response to what is felt to be a need for these diffuse and often unrelated aspects of radiology to be gathered together in a compact and concise form. It is intended to be both a ready reference to any problem that may suddenly arise and perhaps to stimulate interest amongst radiologists and forensic practitioners concerning the current medico-legal status of radiology.

Most of the material in this book is not new, but hitherto it has been distributed widely amongst the world literature, often lurking under some obscure title or in some exotic journal. It is felt that by consolidating this information under one cover, its accessibility will be greatly increased. To the best of our knowledge, no similar book has previously appeared, certainly not in the English language. In addition to this reference material, there are some original observations on the significance of hyoid fractures and on the reliability of identification from radiographs of individual bones.

The authors have been at pains to avoid any territorial limitations of the applicability of the contents of the book. This disadvantage tends to occur in most medico-legal publications, as the legal systems of different countries vary so widely. Though most of the examples quoted herein are either British or American in origin, the forensic pathology and the broad principles of the malpractice issues should have fairly universal application.

Particular thanks are due to Dr D. K. Whittaker, Senior Lecturer in Oral Biology at the Welsh National School of Medicine, who is recognized by the Home Office as the forensic odontologist for Wales. He has kindly provided the section on the radiological aspects of his subject, which is so specialized as to be outside the main-stream of general medical or forensic expertise.

We trust that the book will fill the traditional 'long-felt want' as virtually every radiologist is sooner or later confronted with a medico-legal problems. This ready reference may well provide the advice he requires.

K.T.E.
B.K.

Acknowledgements

The authors would like to offer their grateful thanks to the following for cases and films included in this work—Dr O. G. Williams (Swansea), Dr F. S. Grebbel (Belfast), Dr R. K. Levick (Sheffield), Dr Roy Astley (Birmingham), Dr M. G. E. Greensmith (Wrexham) and to many consultant radiologists and paediatricians in Cardiff.

1 Medico-legal radiology an historical introduction

The forensic use of X-rays followed hard upon the heels of Roentgen's original discoveries—one of the first on record took place in a terraced house in a Lancashire textile town.

In January 1896, a letter appeared in the *Manchester Guardian* from Arthur Schuster, Professor of Physics at Owens College, Manchester, drawing attention to the medical potential of Roentgen's work. Professor Schuster had just received from Roentgen the original paper and photographs about the discovery of X-rays, and his letter was the first really authoritative pronouncement on the exciting new advance.

Within a few months, Schuster and his colleagues were involved in a dramatic ballistics investigation which must surely be the first recorded forensic use of radiology in locating metallic objects in a criminal case.

A Mrs Hartley was shot in the head by her husband, Hargreaves Hartley who then drowned himself in the Leeds and Liverpool Canal. His wife, Elizabeth Ann Hartley, was aged 22 and a loom operator like her husband. He fired four shots from a pistol at close range into her head on 23 April 1896, exactly 3 months after the translation of Roentgen's paper had appeared in *Nature*.

Three days later, a photographer from Burnley made an unsuccessful attempt to take an X-ray of her head, as she had survived the shooting and lay conscious in bed at her home at 20 North Street, Nelson, a typical small terraced house in the working-class district of the mill town.

Dr William Little, a local general practitioner, then asked Professor Schuster to try to locate the bullets by

Roentgen ray. Schuster was unwell and sent his assistants, C. H. Lees and A. Stanton on 29 April. The first exposure was said to have taken 1 hour and the second 70 minutes! Professor (later Sir) Arthur Schuster developed the plates himself and found three of the bullets in her cranium. On 2 May, he went himself to Nelson and took another plate which revealed the fourth missile. Unfortunately Mrs Hartley died on 9 May, being too weak to undergo any attempt at surgical removal.

There is neither a record of a post-mortem nor any photographs, but it is known that the bullets were beyond the reach of a surgical probe. The apparatus needed for this domiciliary forensic exercise was formidable. The team took to the house 3 glass Crooke's tubes (2 as spares), the high tension coil and glass photographic plates. All these fragile objects had to be transported over rough cobblestones by a horse-drawn cab from the railway station. There was no mains electricity in the narrow streets and the local Nelson Corporation supplied storage batteries to provide the power for the cumbersome apparatus, which would have had to be assembled in the tiny bedroom.

The Mayor and Town Clerk of Nelson were amongst those attending the 'experiment' as it was called in the *Nelson and Colne Express*, which printed a blow-by-blow account of the whole procedure. It must have been a harrowing experience, as Stanton, one of the assistants, suffered a nervous breakdown afterwards, directly attributed to the radiography of the mutilated and dying woman.

In principle, nothing has altered in those 84 years, apart from the complexity of the equipment, and the experience of the radiologists. Though forensic radiographs are now rarely taken in the upstairs bedrooms of small terraced houses, the indications and usefulness of the procedure and the broad principles of the technique remain the same as they did on that nineteenth-century day in a North Country mill town, when forensic radiology was born. (Schuster, Nora (1968)

2 Radiology in identification

The use of radiology in investigating the identity of post-mortem skeletal structures is often confused in general textbooks with the ordinary anatomical measurement and examination of bones. In many instances, radiography may add nothing to visual inspection and indeed may sometimes not be as useful, because exact measurements of bone dimensions, gained by the use of an osteometric board and calipers, may be more accurate than measurement of images on radiographs which may contain some degree of enlargement. Caution must therefore be used in advocating the use of radiography on a haphazard basis, where it is not likely to add to the knowledge gained by anatomical investigation and measurement. However, there are frequent occasions where radiography is of considerable use, and on some occasions it is indispensable. Where the intact body is concerned—whether dead or occasionally even alive—radiological examination may be the only practical means of examining the skeleton for purposes of identity. There are similar advantages where partly decomposed material is to be examined or where some suspicious amorphous mass, frequently recovered from mass disasters, may contain skeletal material.

The use of radiological examination in the identification of skeletal structures fall into three main groups:

(a) The primary anatomical investigation to determine whether bones actually are present, whether or not they are human and basic features such as age, sex and stature. Where no previous radiographs are available, this may be the limit of possible investigation.

(b) The comparison of two sets of radiographs, one obtained from a potential matching subject from previous films taken for diagnostic purposes, the other set being taken at the time of the investigation. Here, the object is to match the visual appearances and dimensions of various anatomical landmarks and structures in order to establish or eliminate a perfect match.

(c) Another very important use of radiography is in the detection of old and recent injuries involving skeletal structures, including bone deformities, congenital defects and disease processes, all of which may aid in the identification of the unknown subjects. This necessitates previous knowledge of such an abnormality in the putative matching person, but differs from the comparison between ante-mortem and post-mortem radiographs mentioned above, as there may be no ante-mortem radiological evidence available. Even without such radiographs, the correspondence of certain abnormalities may be extremely useful in the partial or even total correlation between the skeletal remains and a clinical description of the lesion in the potential match.

Returning to what may be termed 'comparison radiography', the essential process is the visual matching (with exact measurement if necessary) of two sets of radiographs, one obtained from some previous clinical diagnostic episode, the other being taken at the time of investigation. Naturally, this process is usually performed on post-mortem material, but there have been occasions where the identity of a living person needs to be proved. The subject may be comatose, amnesic, mentally deranged or, on a very few occasions, identity may be deliberately withheld or falsified in connection with some criminal offence or even inpersonation for monetary or other reasons.

The vast majority of cases requiring skeletal identification involve the finding of a dead body, either intact, partly or wholly skeletalized. The necessity for identification is obvious and is not necessarily related to crime. Relatives of a missing person are usually anxious to have the identity of discovered remains proved or eliminated. The coroner or medical examiner requires all possible information as to identity, and where there is suspicion or evidence of crime, then the matter is of paramount importance to law enforcement authorities. Some parts of the skeleton are much more useful than others for comparison radiography and indeed some parts of the body are of little or no use. However, by the extension of techniques for multi-parameter comparison studies, even the most unlikely material may become more useful in future.

By far the most helpful area of the body for comparison radiography is the skull. Apart from the teeth and jaws, which will be considered in a separate chapter, the rest of the skull has more characteristic features than any other part of the skeleton.

The skull has featured in recent research into complex multi-dimensional measurements as a means of identity. This specialty of cephalometry has been pursued most closely by Sassouni. Using the skull as a whole, Sassouni developed a technique in which he used left lateral and postero–anterior views to establish exact cephalometric indices. The radiographs were taken in the Broadbent–Bolton Roentgenographic Cephalometer. In an experimental series of almost 500 young adult American males, both white and negro, he took two such sets of records, using the first to simulate the ante-mortem set of films and the second to simulate the post-mortem films.

On the PA film, Sassouni took 24 measurements and calculated the range of variation and the standard of deviation for each. This was done on a sample of 30 subjects. The remainder of the films were measured by two different investigators and the total range of error assessed for each measurement. The ratio between standard deviation and error was calculated and only those in which the ratio was greater than two were retained. Two diameters were eliminated because of duplication. The selected measurements from the PA film were: bigonial breadth, mastoid to apex height, bimaxillary breadth, bizygomatic breadth, maximum cranial breadth, sinus breadth, incisor height and total facial height.

On the lateral film a similar study revealed that 8 measurements were significant: cranial height at 8 cm posterior, 4 cm posterior directly above and 4 cm anterior to the sella; cranial height along nasion–sella 4 cm above and 8 cm above; and total facial height (nasion–menton).

Using these 16 measurements, further standard deviation and error calculations were made and eventually only 5 measurements proved to be critical. These were: length of cranium 4 cm above the nasion–sella line; total facial height (nasion–menton); sinus breadth; bigonial breadth; and bizygomatic breadth.

As the latter 4 were all taken from the PA film, the first measurements were discarded in order to save the trouble and expense of a lateral film. The PA view only was used, employing the total 8 frontal measurements, this being sufficient in Sassouni's view to make a positive identity in every case where there are two films available for comparison. He conducted a computer check on the accuracy and arrived at a 97% correct identification. The 8 measurements are shown in Fig. 2.1. The 3 remaining films could either be identified by further cross-checking, leading to a virtual 100% success rate. Sassouni calculated that with 20 measurements one individual can be identified out of $3\frac{1}{2}$ million subjects.

In later work, Sassouni developed an analysis of individuality employing basic *planes* of reference, taken from lateral cephalometric films. These planes comprised (a) a cranial base plane, (b) a palatal plane, (c) an occlusal (dental) plane and (d) a mandibular base plane. He also employed two basic arcs intercepting the four plantes at determined points, one anterior and one posterior. This technique is claimed to be useful in reconstructing the profile of a skull which is only present in a fragmentary state by extrapolation from the planes and arcs. For further details, the original publications should be consulted (Sassouni, 1955; 1957; 1959).

Another part of the skull has also been suggested as a useful comparison region for identity studies. This is the sphenoid bone and its various components, used by Voluter in his 'V-tests'. Voluter claims that the area of the sella is of particular importance because of its protected situation, and thus it is one of the last areas to

Fig. 2.1. Tracing of
postero–anterior skull
radiograph showing selected
measurements (after Sassouni):
(1) bigonial breadth, (2)
mastoid to apex height, (3)
bimaxillary breadth, (4)
bizygomatic breadth, (5)
maximum cranial breadth, (6)
sinus breadth, (7) incisor
height, and (8) total facial
height.

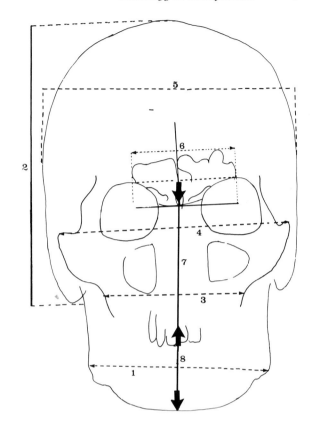

be damaged or destroyed by destructive processes such as fire, extreme violence or decay. The V-test takes notice of the form and volume of the pituitary fossa, the angle formed by the clivus and the anterior cranial base (The 'sella angle or Sattlewinkel') in craniometry, the size and shape of this sphenoidal sinus and the osseous structure and extent and position of air cells around the sella. Voluter claims that these points are as unique as fingerprints when used as matching criteria in ante-mortem and post-mortem films (Voluter, 1960).

Several workers have used cephalic radiography to calculate other dimensions which may well have unique and individual properties, such as the calcula-tion of the endocranial dimensions, the derivation of an encephalic index and the estimation of an endocranial volume, for which the work of Mollison (1925), Neuert (1931) and Haas (1952) must be studied.

FRONTAL SINUS RADIOGRAPHY IN IDENTIFICATION

Less complicated techniques were suggested many years before Sassouni's work. In 1921, Schuller pointed out that the frontal sinuses, as observed radiographically, were useful in identification. In 1931, Thomas A. Poole stated that the frontal sinuses of no two persons were alike. This has been amply confirmed since and much has been written upon the use of the frontal sinuses in identity matching, including a monograph by Asherson (1965).

The frontal sinuses appear in the second year of life and increase in size until about the twentieth year of life. Unfortunately, in about 5% of adults no frontal sinuses may be observed radiographically and in a smaller portion, about 1%, they are unilaterial. The sinuses tend to be larger in males than in females, the latter having more numerous and smaller scalloped upper archings. In old age, the walls of the sinuses become thinner and the sinuses appear larger. Also in senile states, the sinuses may communicate with the diploic spaces between the tables of the skull.

In 1927, Culbert and Law presented a case history of identification using frontal sinus patterns, together with certain details of the mastoid process. They claimed a number of points of identity in the mastoid radiographic pattern.

Schüller (1943) recommends orienting the head or skull in the 'forehead–nose position' for radiography, with the axis of the tube level with the supra-orbital margins. On comparing the films, special notice is taken of the upper borders of the sinus which shows scalloped arches, any partial or complete septa, the line of the frontal septum and any supra-orbital air cells. His actual recommendations for comparison are given below and in Fig. 2.2.

'The following are the bony details to be observed in the radiograph: the line of the frontal septum; the upper

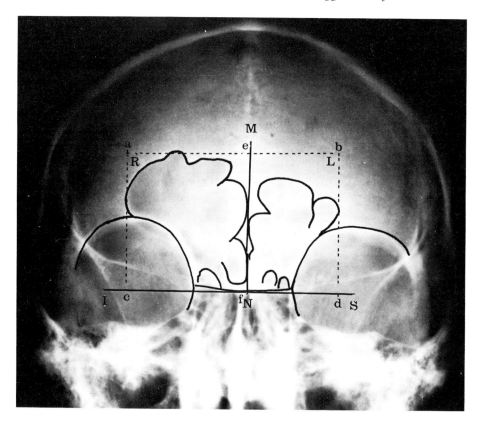

Fig. 2.2. The outline of the frontal sinuses and orbits and measurements of the frontal sinuses (after Fuller).

border of the frontal sinus; partial septa; supraorbital cells. In the skull, the line of the septum deviates from the mid-line towards the right side; the upper border is scalloped with two arcades on the right and three on the left frontal sinus; one partial septum is present between the medial and the two lateral arcades of the left frontal sinus; two cells are seen in the lower half of the left frontal area, the lateral cell, marked by one cross, representing a supraorbital extension, the medial cell, marked by two crosses, representing a *bulla frontalis* of the ethmoid.

'In order to measure the diameters of the frontal sinuses I use a simple construction—namely, a vertical line corresponding to the median sagittal section of the forehead (MN), a horizontal line (IS) corresponding to the projection of the *jugum (planum) sphenoidale*, one rectangle (R + L) framing the upper border and the two lateral borders of both combined frontal sinuses (abcd) and another rectangle (L) framing the larger sinus (ebdf).

'The line MN can be determined readily in the great majority of cases, because the dense line of the frontal crest is generally easily seen in the X-ray picture corresponding to the attachment of the *falx cerebri* on the inner surface of the vertical plate. Sometimes the outlines of a narrow groove are visible; this is the anterior part of the longitudinal sinus. A persistent frontal suture may indicate the midline, or the rim of the *crista galli* facilitates its recognition. Finally, the position of the characteristic shadows representing ossifications along the *falx cerebri* or calcifications of the pineal body may serve the same purpose.

'The line IS is drawn perpendicularly to the midline. It represents the level of the *jugum (planum) sphenoidale*, which forms the roof of the body of the sphenoid bone on the floor of the anterior cranial fossa, just behind the *lamina cribosa*. This line of the *jugum sphenoidale* lies in the same horizontal level as the bottom of the frontal sinus in the majority of cases, as it is seen in profile pictures of the anterior cranial fossa. In the standard forehead–nose view, the projection of the *jugum sphenoidale* is always visible as a straight or slightly curved outline, which crosses the projection of the medial border and/or the medial wall of the orbit. The line IS joining these points perpendicular to MN, indicates the level of the floor of the frontal sinuses. The horizontal line IS forms the base for the construction of the rectangular frames of the two combined frontal sinuses (R + L) and the larger left sinus (L); a horizontal line is drawn through the highest point of the left frontal sinus, and three vertical lines are drawn, two along the most lateral points of the left and the right sinus, and one along the right border of the left sinus. The exact measurements are taken of the width (ab) of the rectangular frame for both combined sinuses, the width (eb) of the rectangle for the left sinus and the height (ef) of the rectangle for the left sinus. These three measurements, combined with the description of the frontal septa, of the arches of the upper border of the frontal sinuses and of the separate cells in the supraorbital region, should allow one to identify the frontal sinus of each individual skull. It is obvious that the three measurements are sufficient as fundamentals for the classification of large numbers of cases and may be used as the basis of a filing system for the X-ray pictures.'

Asherson (1965) recommends a standard procedure for visualizing the frontal sinuses radiographically, by taking films in the occipito–mental plane, which he points out is a rapid, simple and standard procedure in the investigation of the nasal accessory sinuses (Fig. 2.3). If the occipito–mental exposure is accurately posed, Asherson states that there is always a constant outline of the frontal sinuses, suitable for comparison. He points out that the frontal sinuses are usually radiographed in the special occipito–frontal position, an additional exposure which can also be used to secure a frontal sinus print. The occipito–mental and the occipito–frontal views of the frontal sinuses are by no means identical, and frequently differ markedly. Asherson quotes Pancoast, who states: 'The frontal sinuses are peculiarly amenable to roentgen examination and several positions are utilized—the Caldwell (occipito–mental) and the Wallers (occipito–frontal).' Asherson states that long experience of viewing the frontal sinuses in the standard occipito–mental view has impressed him with the precision and accuracy of the positioning of the head when this exposure is made, so that films taken by different radiographers, or the same radiographer at intervals of time, reveal identical and superimposable views of the frontal sinuses.

According to Asherson, a template of the shape of the frontal sinuses can be outlined in ink on a photographic contact print made from the negative film or by tracing the outline onto tracing paper. Such a template can be filed and be used to compare the radiological shape and size of the frontal sinuses in any subsequent identification procedure. Another method suggested is that used by French investigators (Turpin & Tisserand, 1942) where the film image is projected onto a cardboard screen. The outline of the frontal sinuses is marked onto the cardboard and then cut out

Fig. 2.3. (a) Occipito–mental view (ante-mortem). (b) Same projection at autopsy. The outline of the frontal sinuses and bone detail in the antra are identical.

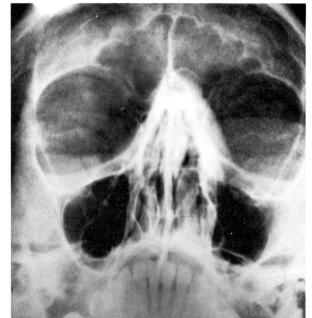

(a)

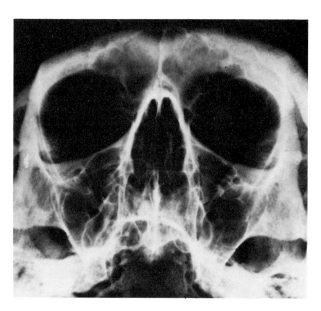

(b)

to shape. By weighing the templates, a comparison of the total area can be made for each case. However, this method is open to criticism, as frontal sinuses of different shape from different persons may fortuitously have the same surface area. Asherson states categorically that there is no identity of the frontal sinus prints in twins, whether identical or non-identical.

Oksanen and Kormano (1978) claim that in addition to the other identifying features in radiography of the skull, the vascular grooves of the cranial vault, such as the course of the middle meningeal artery and its branches, may assist in comparing ante-mortem with post-mortem films.

The potential use of cranial radiography in identification became so obvious that in 1953, Thorne and Thyberg suggested that a form of 'mass miniature radiography' should be employed on a large scale as a method of 'prophylactic' identification. In order to test their claims, they took two sets of films, both in the lateral and AP views, at a distance of one metre from 100 children and adults, the films being spaced one month apart. On later comparison of these films they claim that 'it was possible to perform such an identification in all cases without difficulty' using tracings of dimensions, indices and angles. It is said that a similar technique is used for air-crew of the United States Air Force, in order that films may always be on record of frontal sinus patterns, etc., in case identification is later required following an aviation tragedy. It has also been reported that proposals to obtain the same anticipatory films on civilian air-crew have been rejected by the commercial air-crew unions, the basic reason apparently being a reluctance to 'tempt providence'.

Occasionally, comparison radiographs of the skull may yield matching criteria other than anatomical structures. In a homicide case reported by Mann and Fatteh (1968), the exhumed remains of the victim were identified solely by comparison of sets of radiographs which displayed the effects of previous gunshot wounds. The deceased had previously been wounded in the face by a revolver bullet and the consequent fracture-deformity of the zygomatic arch was accepted by the court as being sufficiently accurate proof of comparability in the two sets of films.

WRIST AND HAND RADIOGRAPHY

Bones other than the skull also have their uses in identity by comparison methods. Greulich (1960) studied the radiological features of the wrist and hand, especially the distal radius, distal ulna, carpals, metacarpals and phalanges. He maintained that traits of individuality are established in these bones in late adolescence and remain relatively unchanged until well into the fourth decade. Greulich claimed to be able to differentiate between identical twins on radiographs of the wrist and hand. His techniques showed that it was quite easy to pair right and left hands from amongst a series of mixed wrist–hand radiographs. Greulich also claimed that there were racial differences between American whites, Americans and Japanese Americans. The features he considered were especially the shape and size of the styloid processes of the radius and ulna, the width of the cortices and medullary cavities, the shape and proportions of the phalanges and the trabecular pattern in the shafts.

THORACIC RADIOLOGY

The pattern of ossification in the costal cartilage of the first rib is also useful in identifying two chest radiographs and is used as a practical tool by clinical radiologists on the rare occasions when there is confusion as to the origin of two chest films (King, 1939). It seems that the pattern of ossification in this area is unique though presumably a long interval between the two films might alter the ossification pattern, which progresses with age. Comparison radiographs must be made in similar anatomical positions (Fig. 2.4). The clavicle has also been recommended as a bone with unique radiographic appearances. Sanders *et al.* (1972) reported a case where the only surviving bone was a left clavicle together with some shattered other bones of no use for anatomical examination. Comparison with chest films of a potential match were eventually obtained and a comparison of the minute details of radiographs of the two bones was made. The medial portion of the clavicle furnished a number of identifiable details which were primarily used in the comparison. These included the general configuration, the cortical thickness in various specific areas, the

Fig. 2.4. (a) Localized view of the first left costo-chondral junction taken from an ante-mortem chest radiograph. (b) Excised sternum and first rib showing irregular ossifiation of the costal cartilage. The detail is identical to 2.4(a).

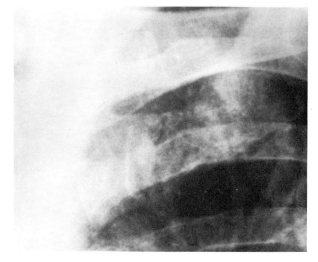

(a)

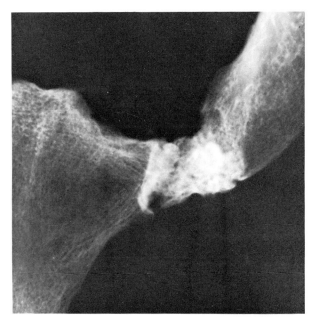

(b)

anatomical variant of a tiny cortical spur on the inferior medial aspect of the bone and specific trabecular pattern and detail. From a technical point of view, it was found that a better picture was obtained from the isolated clavicle if a water bolus was overlaid, rather than a 'bare' exposure made. Although on occasions as in Fig. 2.5 (a–b) it is possible to obtain a direct match—

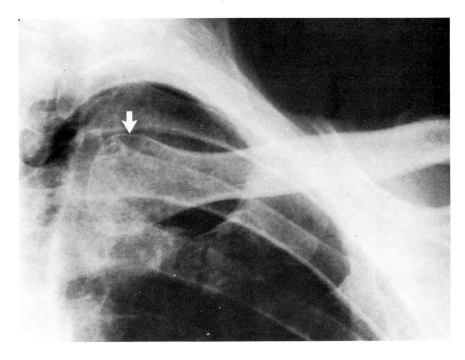

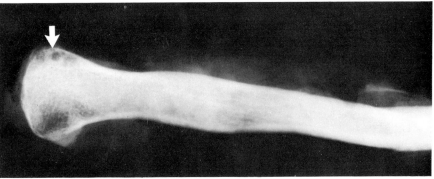

Fig. 2.5. (a) Ante-mortem chest radiograph showing small cysts in the medial end of the clavicle. (b) Radiograph of excised clavicle showing identical appearances.

this is by no means invariable. It is frequently difficult to obtain radiographs in identical anatomical positions and in some cases it is impossible to match the radiographs taken in life with the excised specimen.

Other useful areas of the body include the cervical and thoracic spine and pelvis. In the 'Noronic' disaster in Toronto in 1949, mobile X-ray equipment was used to identify the 24 individuals by using radiographs obtained during life for comparison with autopsy films (Fig. 2.6). Amongst these 24 cases, the skull was used

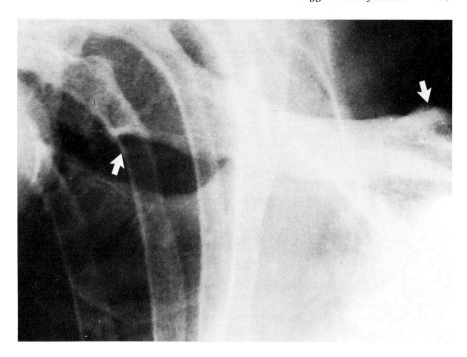

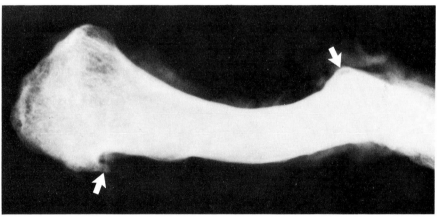

Fig. 2.6. Identification made easy by the presence of a spur of the inferior aspect of the left clavicle medially and a small cyst on its superior aspect laterally.

in 4 cases, the cervical spine in 2, the thoracic spine and chest in 13, the lumbar spine and pelvis in 9 and foot and ankle in 1 (Singleton, 1951; Brown *et al.*, 1952).

COMPARISON RADIOGRAPHY IN ESTABLISHING IDENTITY

Another aspect of comparison radiography in identification depends not upon individual anatomical variations, but upon the matching of specific abnormalities of a variety of types.

Old fractures with deformity, callus formation, angulation and other unique abnormalities which can be compared on two films separated in time, form a vital part of this type of identification. Again, it is naturally essential to have ante-mortem and post-mortem films available, the former almost invariably coming from clinical sources during the treatment of the condition which led to the deformity or from some other unassociated diagnostic radiograph.

Several examples can be quoted from the authors' experience. A skeletalized body was discovered in January 1977, with sufficient soft tissue to indicate that death had occurred within the previous year. The usual anatomical investigation revealed that it was a middle-aged male of a certain stature. Police records provided three or four missing persons where the sex, age, stature and time factor were compatible. The ribs of the skeleton showed callus formation on several ribs on each side and one of the potential matches had a history of a chest injury in July 1976. Films were obtained from the hospital where this person was treated and an exact match was made between the position of the callus and the fractures revealed on the clinical film (Fig. 2.7).

In another instance, a badly decomposed and incomplete body was washed up on the foreshore of the Bristol Channel, the almost bare skull showing the typical features of acromegaly. In addition there was a small penetrating defect in the centre of the forehead communicating with the frontal sinus. A raised, smooth bone edge around this defect indicated that it was an ante-mortem lesion and not post-mortem damage. During 3 months police investigation, several possible matching candidates were presented, but eventually one was found who had a history of a head injury from a traffic accident 7 years previously. The

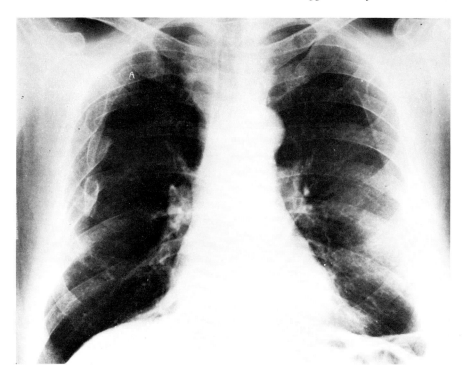

Fig. 2.7. Old fracture of some of the ribs in the right side. Identical fractures located at autopsy.

old clinical notes indicated that there had been a penetrating wound of the forehead. The skull films were traced, the presence of mild acromegaly was confirmed and not only did the forehead defect match the skull, but radiographs proved beyond any doubt that the outlines of the frontal sinuses were exactly comparable.

In the latter case, acromegaly was one factor which was helpful in the identification and other bony diseases may sometimes offer similar assistance. Paget's disease of the skull is one that is perhaps too common to be more useful than a suggestive pointer. An isolated femur, again washed up on the shores of the Bristol Channel, showed a marked increase in weight and density and radiology confirmed the presence of a condition resembling the Albers–Schoenberg (marble bone) disease. Unfortunately, no possible matching candidate was ever put forward so the presence of this condition was of no use. This underlines the absolute necessity of a potential matching candidate before such comparisons can be made, assuming that ante-mortem films can be retrieved on the putative 'identities'.

Many instances of trauma, disease processes and congenital anomalies can be thought of, which may provide total or partial comparison identity.

In a complicated homicide case, the body of a woman (recovered from a river after having been submerged by means of weights for about 6 weeks) was the subject of an intense police investigation, as the cause of death was strangulation. When a short-list of matching potential victims was further investigated, there was disagreement between relatives as to the identity from visual appearances of the now decomposing body. The putative match had previously had a cholecystectomy and the body had no gall bladder, and had an upper abdominal operation scar. There had also been a traffic accident one year before death and scars upon the knees corresponded with records in the hospital notes. From a radiological point of view the prize finding was the presence of a sesamoid bone in the left Achilles tendon, visible on the clinical films taken for the leg injury and confirmed on post-mortem radiography. Ossification in the Achilles tendon generally develops after trauma, though it can occur without previous trauma (Kohler). This rather rare condition, combined with the other factors, made identity absolute and contributed to the eventual conviction for murder of the husband—a detective-inspector of police!

The presence of foreign bodies observed radiographically may also provide matching evidence against ante-mortem films. Numerous examples can be quoted, from joint prostheses, femoral pins and plates to metal sutures and surgical clips. Foreign bodies introduced traumatically may also be revealed, such as shrapnel or bullet fragments, or from the effects of industrial or traffic accidents.

In children and young persons, there may be a unique pattern of arrested growth lines (Harris's lines) in the metaphyses which may be matched by careful comparison of their spacing and prominence. Gordon and Ross (1977) have pointed out that if chondrogenesis occurs more slowly than normal, even if only for a short time, a dense plate in the metaphysis may result. This may be produced by an acute illness, nutritional deficiency or following irradiation. They are most commonly seen in the long bones such as the distal end of the femur, both ends of the ulna and the distal end of the radius, they may also be seen in the cuboid bones. Harris's lines remain at the same distance from the centre of the shaft as they were when formed. They may eventually fragment and fade, and this occurs more rapidly the younger the child is at the time of their formation. They may also persist into late adult life. In a case shown by Gordon and Ross (1977) an additional Harris's line developed between two films taken at nine-monthly intervals. The presence of Harris's lines, although of importance, become progressively less useful with the passage of time. They may, however, be a useful addition to the general comparison of limb bones from the outline, cortical thickness and cancellous pattern, but the films from which comparisons are made should not be separated by too great a time interval if exact correspondence is to be gained, as osseous remodelling may be relatively rapid and extensive in actively growing bones.

Where two sets of films are available, separated in time by a period which is unlikely to introduce errors in ageing, then if the positions are standard enough to avoid significant errors from different angulation or magnification, the experienced radiologist can frequently satisfy himself that the films came from the same person by matching of numerous points of reference, including the superimposition of various anatomical landmarks and by a multiplicity of similarities in the bone structure itself. Where a pelvic view or a skull is available, then the experienced viewer may trust to his visual matching rather than resort to the complex measurements as described by Sassouni. This less formalized approach is not to decry the careful mathematical computations of the cephalometrists, but may be employed with a correspondingly smaller degree of certainty where sophisticated measurements cannot be taken. These visual comparisons are also very useful in *excluding* identity as where the two sets of films are within technical limits of comparability, then an absence of matching can frequently be diagnosed at a glance.

RADIOGRAPHY IN THE ESTABLISHMENT OF GENERAL GROUPINGS IN IDENTITY

In the previous section the use of radiography was discussed in the establishment of the unique identity of a given individual by comparison of ante-mortem and post-mortem films. Radiography also has an important role in assisting in establishing general groupings in identity. In other words, where there is no opportunity to specifically identify the individual by comparison of two films, the identity must be narrowed down as much as possible by an evaluation of species, sex, age, race and stature.

Where bony remains are recovered, the first necessity is to determine whether they are human or animal. In fact, on some occasions a preliminary decision is needed as to whether or not they are actually bones. In one case known to the authors, a perfectly formed human clavicle turned out to be a plaster-of-Paris replica. In archaeological work, even stones may sometimes bear a remarkable likeness to fragmental fossil material, and in both these instances radiography would immediately solve the doubt.

Species determination

Returning to the species determination, most of the examination will turn upon a knowledge of human and animal anatomy where radiography may not play any significant part. Where the fragments are too small for any anatomical examination then recourse must be made to serology, if the bones are recent enough to have retained sufficient immunological activity.

Where bones are found in association with soft tissue—often decomposed—then radiology may be a more convenient, rapid and accurate method of determining the presence or absence of human skeletal material, without the laborious and offensive task of removing the soft tissue. In some cases with criminal connotations, destructive dissection methods may not be possible in the early stages of examination and radiological examination will provide a rapid, non-destructive and convenient method of revealing the bony anatomy. One well-known case in the United Kingdom—similar to several cases in North America—concerned the finding of what appeared to be a human hand with soft tissue attached. On further examination this turned out to be a paw of a bear, which when partly decomposed held a striking anatomical resemblance to a human hand. In these cases, the radiological findings would immediately reveal the difference.

Determination of sex

When the remains are confirmed as human, the sex of the person is probably the next most important factor. Once again, visual anatomical examination and measurements are often sufficient to provide the answer, assuming that sufficient skeletal material is available. The skull, pelvis and femora are naturally the most useful for this purpose and radiological examination does not play any important role in such an examination. However, a certain number of cases, especially where the material is incomplete, will not provide a clear-cut decision as to sex, even in post-pubertal skeletons. Before puberty, sexual characteristics are slight or absent, both anatomically and radiologically. Where post-pubertal material gives uncertain results, then radiology can sometimes assist in giving accurate pelvic dimensions from which certain formulae can be applied, with more accurate results than direct visual measurement of the bones.

Though sexing of immature material is difficult, Reynolds (1945) made radiological studies of the bony pelvic girdle in early infancy in an effort to detect sex differences at this age. Reynolds made measurements on the radiographs of 46 boys and 49 girls (American white race) during the first year of age, taking serial films at birth, 1, 3, 6, 9 and 12 months. A complex set of measurements were taken and indices of proportions derived from them. The details should be obtained from the original paper. Reynolds's conclusions on sex differences in the first post-natal year included the observation that there were significant differences in that boys lead in pelvis height, ilium breadth and ischio–iliac space. Girls have greater bi-ischial breadth, pubis length, breadth of greater sciatic notch, relative inlet breadth and anterior segment index. He also found that critical ratios of sex differences showed a slight tendency to become smaller with age. The general pattern of sex differences in the pelvis as shown by Reynolds's study seems to favour the hypothesis that boys are larger in measurement relating to the outer structure of the pelvis while girls are larger in measurement relating to the inner structures of the pelvis, including a relatively larger inlet.

Reynolds (1947) also studied radiological differences in the pelvis of male and female children between 2 and 9 years. These results showed that girls showed higher intercorrelations in measurements at 3 years than did boys, which was contrary to his findings in the first year of life where a tendency towards higher intercorrelations was shown by the boys. There were significant sex differences at various age levels, the details of which should be sought in the original publication. Critical ratios of sex differences are larger at 22 months than at any of the succeeding age levels to 9 years. Again there appears to be a tendency for sex differences to become less pronounced with age in the pre-pubertal period. As in the infant study, the measurements of girls tend to be more variable than the measurements of boys. As in the infant group, this older study also indicated that the pelvic measurements in boys are larger in relation to the exterior of the pelvis, while the female pelvis tends to have a relatively larger inlet.

Thomas and Greulich (1940) also used radiology for pelvimetry in order to develop anatomical ratios for various pelvic sexual characteristics. Whether these means are an advantage or a convenience over anatomical measurements is a matter for discussion, but obviously considerable regard must be paid to any magnification factor involved in translating radiological sizes into true anatomical measurement. Where ratios are being used, perhaps this difference is of less importance.

Determination of age

While radiography plays relatively little part in sex determination, except as a substitute or adjunct for direct measurement, its role in age determination is of vital importance.

In the identification of fetuses, infants and young persons, the appearance of ossification centres and the progress of growth as measured by epiphyseal development and eventual fusion are vital in the determination of age up to the early part of the third decade.

The development of teeth, both deciduous and permanent dentition, is also of vital importance in the ageing of skeletal material, but this will be considered separately in the chapter on dental radiology.

The use of radiology in detecting and evaluating ossification centres and epiphyseal development depends upon the use of published tables. Unfortunately various tables give different time scales for the same bones and it is important to use data which are as comparable as possible with the supposed origin of the remains under examination. This refers to ethnic, geographical and temporal criteria, as all these factors may make an appreciable difference to the timing of the various osseous events. Naturally, sexual differentiations must be achieved first, if at all possible, as there are definite differences in sexual development of these ostological time markers.

The tables of Francis *et al.* (1939) are well known as convenient data records, but others are available such as the radiographic atlases of Greulich and Pyle (1959) and Pyle and Hoerr (1955).

Certain markers appear in a sequence from early childhood onwards: before the eruption of the permanent teeth at about 6 years of age (for example), ossification sites in the vertebrae are of some use. The axis (second cervical) vertebra consists of 4 separate centres until about the age of 3 years, there being two lateral portions constituting the arch, the body and the dens or odontoid process. Coincidental with the eruption of all the deciduous teeth, the two portions of the arch of this vertebra unite posteriorly.

At about 6 years, when the first permanent molars erupt, the anterior part of the axis vertebra begin to fuse and also the two halves of the arch of the axis (first cervical) vertebra unite posteriorly.

After the second permanent molars have erupted, about the age of 12, the major epiphyses begin to unite and this progressive union goes on throughout the second decade. The times of epiphyseal union differ in each sex, girls tending to fuse before boys, though the variation is by no means standard. Again radiological averages must be consulted for the sequence of union, some constructed from data by McKern and Stewart (1957).

The final union is usually that at the sternal end of the clavicle, which usually fuses in the early or mid-twenties, but which may be as early as 18 years or even as late as 30 years.

The times of fusion of epiphyses with the metaphysis is a more variable criterion than the appearances of the ossification centres in fetal and infant life. In using tabular data, it is usual to take the middle point of the range of known times of fusion, as stated for the clavicle. Thus three dates can be set for each epiphysis, the earliest, the latest and the median time unless no exact age can be set with certainty. However, where a number of centres are investigated, some degree of correlation usually appears, though it can be said that early fusion in one epiphysis in a given individual might well be part of a general early tendency to fusion in other centres in that same individual.

Another difficulty, especially in younger material where some epiphyses are a long way in time from fusion, is that extended post-mortem changes with drying of the skeleton may lead to complete separation of the epiphysis, so that they are frequently lost when the remains are recovered. This of course indicates that the age of fusion had not yet been reached, but the opportunity has been lost to estimate how near or far from fusion date the development had reached.

A major contribution to the study of epiphyseal

union was made by Stevenson (1924) who recognized four states of fusion: no union, beginning union, recent union and complete union. This, however, was an anatomical distinction rather than a radiological one and even though the two are naturally synchronous.

McKern and Stewart offer five degrees of epiphyseal union (0–4) which can be correlated with radiological appearances. Todd (1930) devised nine consecutive radiological stages as follows:

(i) The period when diaphysial and epiphysial bone approximate each other but as yet show no intimate relation, the adjacent surfaces being ill-defined and composed of cancellous tissue.

(ii) The obscuration of the adjacent surfaces by their transformation into thick, hazy zones.

(iii) The clearing of the haze and appearance of a fine delimiting surface of more condensed tissue shown on the roentgenogram as a fine white line.

(iv) The billowing of adjacent surfaces.

(v) The adjacent surfaces with reciprocal outlines which are parallel to each other.

(vi) The narrowing of the gap between adjacent surfaces.

(vii) The commencement of union when the fine white billowed outlines break up.

(viii) The union complete though recent and appearing on the naked bone as a fine red line.

(ix) The perfected union with continuity of trabeculae from shaft to epiphysis.

Krogman (1962) prefers to examine the bone rather than the radiograph and maintains that on a film, the scar of recent union (the maintenance of radiographic opacity at the site of the piled-up calcification adjacent to the epiphyseo-diaphyseal plane) may persist for several years after demonstrable complete union in the bone itself. Krogman disagrees with Keen (Drennan & Keen, 1953) who stated that 'the periods of fusion indicated by radiographs of the body extremities arc approximately three years earlier than the periods of fusion indicated by anatomical evidence and as given in anatomy textbooks, because epiphyseal lines can remain visible on the bone for a considerable time after the radiographs indicate that the fusion has taken place'. This controversy may be followed in Krogman's book *The Human Skeleton in Forensic Medicine*. In this book there is a great deal of information on the timing of ossification centres and epiphyseal fusion, though such an exhaustive exposition of the literature is given that the conflicting views tend to leave the reader rather bemused as to which advice to accept as the most reliable. Similarly, there is a discussion of racial variation in the ageing of young material, though most available data has been obtained from American Negro and some Indian populations, apart from existing tables on white Caucasians.

After the first few decades of life, ageing of skeletal structures becomes difficult. Radiology plays little part in this aspect of the investigation, compared with its prime importance in the young age group. Some anatomical and dental advances in recent years have made this previously infertile period of life far more amenable to age investigation. Anatomical inspection of the opposing faces of the pubic symphysis, which undergoes continuous remodelling throughout life, has helped to bring a more reliable assessment of age in middle and later life, but radiology plays a much lesser role in this technique than in the investigation of ossification centres and epiphyseal union in early life. However, Todd (1921–30) who developed the pubic symphysis technique, used radiography to investigate the symphysis and described four phases related to age:

(a) 25 years. Fine texture body, undulating surface outline, no definition of extremities, no streak of compacta.
(b) 26–39 years. Average texture body, straight or faintly irregular surface outline, incompletely developed lower extremity, little or no grey streak of compacta.
(c) 40–55 years. Average texture body, a straight or irregular ventral outline, a well-developed lower extremity and fairly dense grey streak of compacta.
(d) 55 or more years. Open texture body, an angular

lower extremity, a dense grey streak of compacta broken into patches marking the ventral margins.

Todd suggests that a really undulating outline with no definition of extremities and no grey streak of compacta, with a finely textured body, cannot occur later than 25 years. A straight or faintly marked irregular outline with an incompletely developed lower extremity, little or no grey streak and a fine or average textured bone defines the age as between 25 and 39 years. A well-developed lower extremity with a straight or irregular outline of the ventral face, a fairly dense grey streak and an average textured body suggests 40–55 years. A dense grey streak of outline broken into patches with an angular lower extremity and an open-textured body indicates an age of 55 or more. A series of radiographs illustrating these features is shown in Fig. 2.8. The work of Todd was later developed and refined by McKern and Stewart, but their methods were almost totally anatomical and had no radiological content.

Some apparently significant research has been carried out in the field of estimating personal age, using the progressive resorption and remodelling of cancellous bone in the upper ends of long-limb bones (Fig. 2.9). Schranz (1959) described the apparent ascent of the medullary cavity of the humerus towards the surgical neck of the bone. This can be studied by longitudinal section, but more conveniently and non-destructively by radiology. The medullary cavity is said to approach the surgical neck in the fifth decade and by the sixth and seventh decades moves up to the epiphyseal line.

Schranz described the age sequence as follows, both by anatomical and radiological examination:

15–16 years: metaphysis (growing end of shaft) still cartilaginous.
17–18 years: incipient union; diaphyseal internal structures still ogival.

Fig. 2.8. Variations in the symphysis pubis with age. Note that the symphysis pubis in females is affected by previous pregnancy.

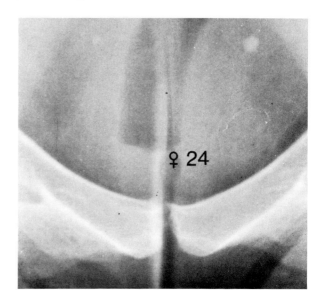

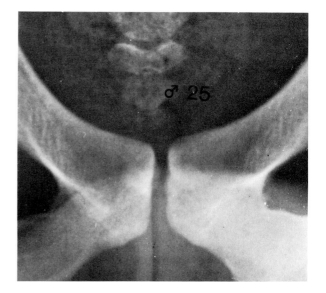

Fig 2.8 continued

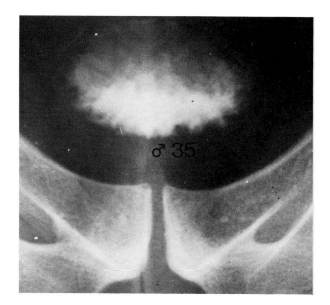

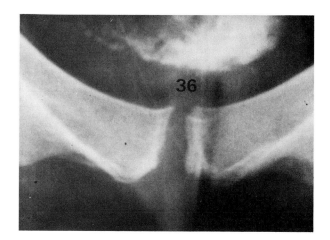

Fig 2.8 continued

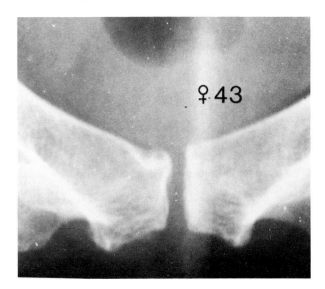

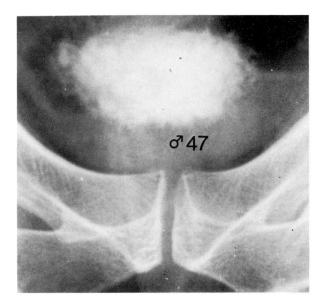

Fig 2.8 continued

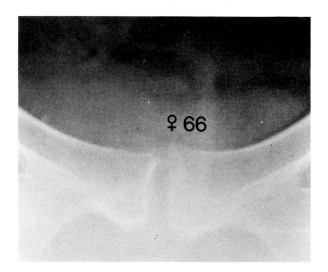

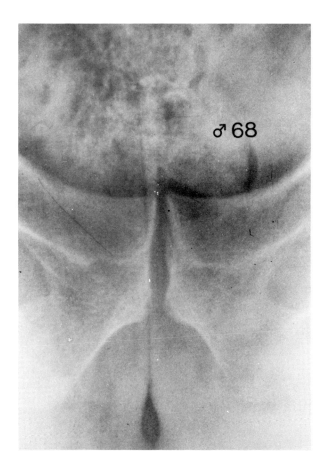

Fig 2.8 continued

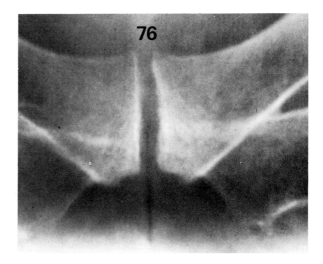

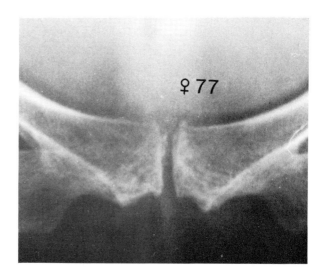

Fig. 2.9. The upper end of the
humerus in various age groups.
Although there are variations
of the configuration with age
these are often not clear cut
and would clearly be affected by
disease in the shoulder joint.

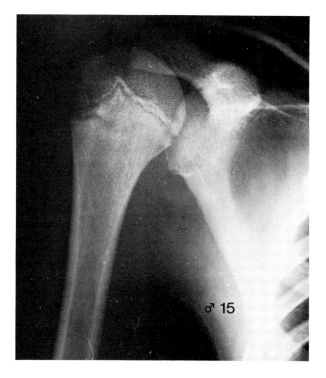

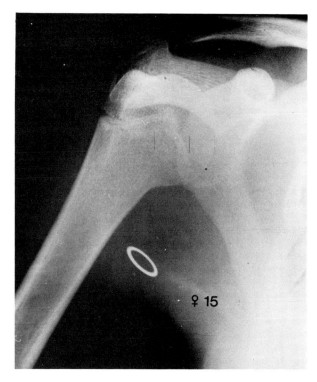

Fig 2.9 continued

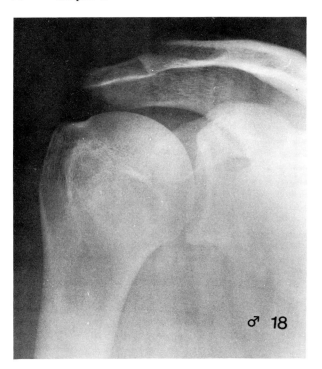

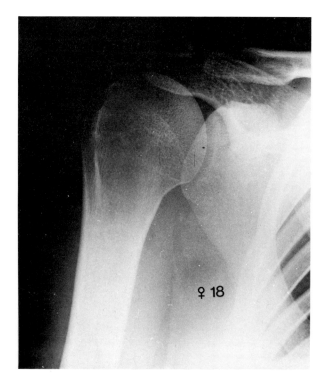

Fig 2.9 continued

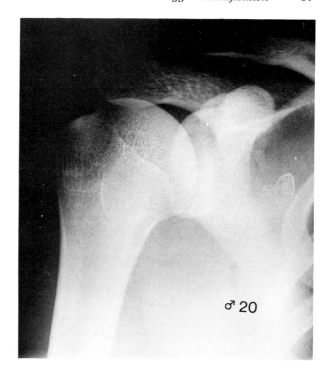

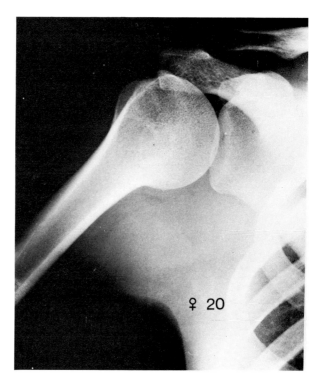

Fig 2.9 continued

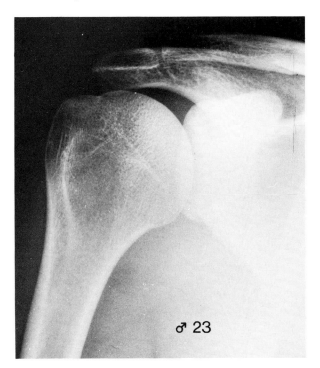

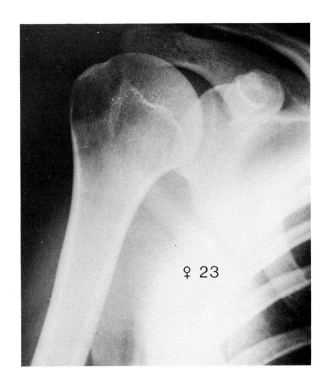

Fig 2.9 continued

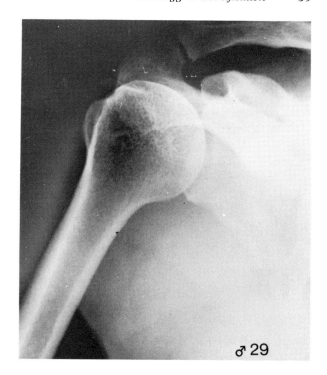

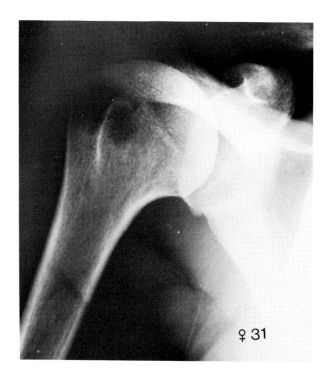

Fig 2.9 continued

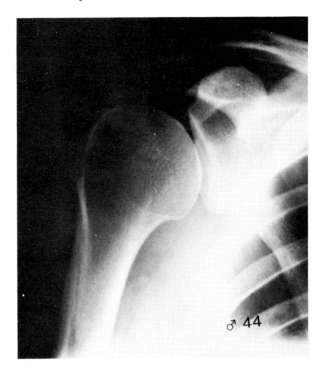

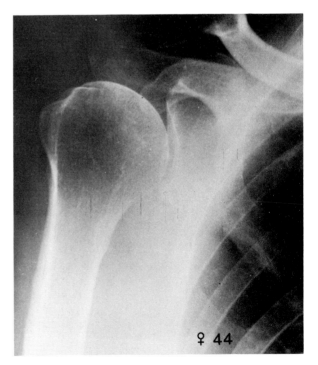

Fig 2.9 continued

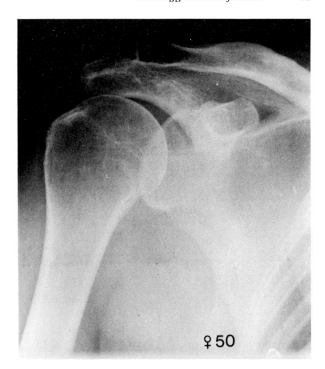

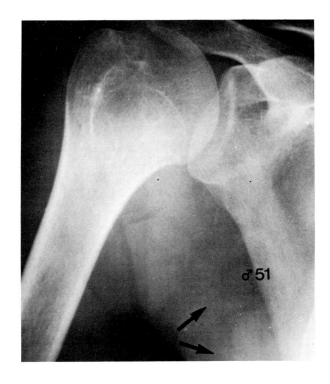

Fig 2.9 continued

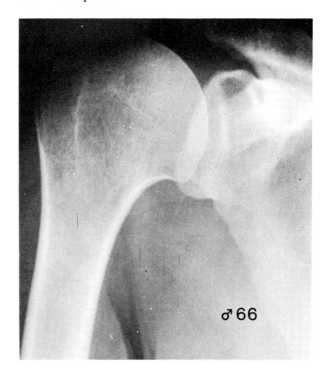

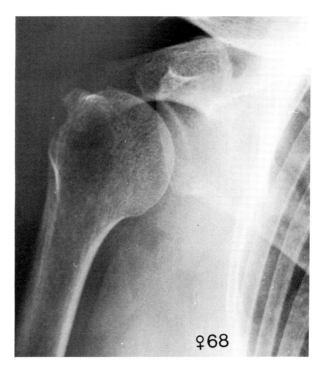

Fig 2.9 continued

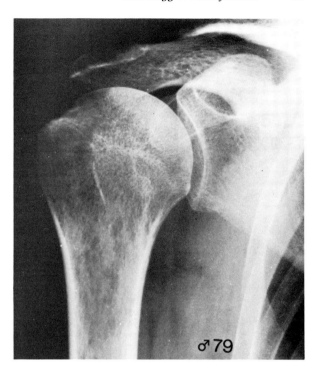

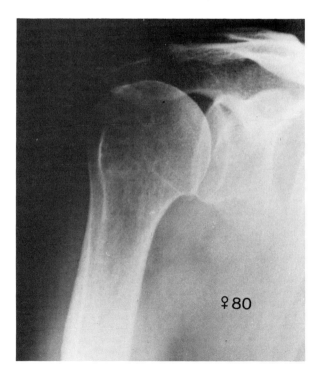

19–20 years: union nearly complete; internal structure of epiphysis is radial, of diaphysis ogival.

21–22 years: union complete, with few traces of cartilage still on external surface; internal structures as in 19–20 years.

23–25 years: development of metaphysis complete; internal structure of epiphysis no longer quite radial, of diaphysis still ogival; medullary cavity is far from the surgical neck.

26–30 years: radial nature of internal structure of epiphysis is fading; that of diaphysis still ogival; medullary cavity not to surgical neck yet.

31–40 years: internal structure of epiphysis no longer radial; that of diaphysis more columniform; most superior part of medullary cavity is near surgical neck.

41–50 years: columniform structure of diaphysis is discontinuous; cone of medullary cavity is up to surgical neck; between the cone and the epiphyseal line lacunae may occur.

51–60 years: pea-sized lacunae show on the major tubercle.

61–70 years: outer surface of the bone is rough; cortex is thin; diaphyseal internal structure is irregular; medullary cavity is up to epiphyseal line; bean-sized lacunae occur in major tubercle—the head shows transparency.

75 + years: external surface of the bone is rough; major tubercle has lost its prominence; cortex is thin; little spongy tissue remains in the medullary cavity; epiphysis (head) very fragile, with increasing transparency.

In all this the female has an age priority of 2 years at puberty, 5 years at maturity, and 7–10 years in the senium. The femur, Schranz says, does not show such distinctive age changes as does the humerus.

Radiological estimation of age in fetal material. As the necessity for determining the age of fetal material is almost always post-mortem, direct dissection and examination of ossification centres can usually be performed, but again radiology may be not only a more convenient and valuable adjunct but in some cases an obligatory alternative to dissection. Numerous tables of the appearance and progress of fetal ossification centres are available. Useful markers quoted by Tchaperoff (1937) are that the first centre appears about the seventh intra-uterine week. By the ninth week, all cervical and thoracic vertebral bodies, iliac wings and femoral, tibial and fibular shaft centres have appeared. Between the twenty-first and twenty-fifth week, the centre in the valcaneus appears followed by the talus between the twenty-fourth and twenty-eighth weeks. By the thirty-fifth week of intra-uterine life, the lower end of the femur shows an epiphyseal ossification centre and by the thirty-ninth week, the centre for the proximal tibial epiphysis should be visible. Naturally, there is biological variation in all these dates, but it is a useful guide.

Radiological studies covering the fetal period have been made by Flecker (1932) and Hill (1939). These two authors substantially agree on the time scale and a tabular summary is given below.

Noback and Robertson (1951) who carried out both radiological and histological examination of fetal ossification centres indicate that the actual specimen is histologically more reliable than radiological appearances of the same bone. They state that: 'Data obtained from roentgenographs of embryos are of limited value, since the actual formation of a centre precedes the time of its radiological recognition.'

The pre-natal ossification of the pelvis was dealt with in detail by a radiological study made by Francis (1951). He relates the appearances of ossification centres with fetal length in millimetres rather than temporal age.

Krogman's book emphasizes the difficulties of reconciling morphological evidence of epiphyseal union with the radiographic appearances. For example, he says: 'The evaluation of age on bone and via the X-ray film (almost always centering on problems of union) is a mute problem. In the first place, the duration from beginning union to complete union as an individual case, is not well known. In the second place, problems of the persistence if a "scar" of union (at the diaphyseo-

Table 2.1. Appearances of pre-natal ossification centres as determined from radiological surveys by Flecker and by Hill

Lunar month	CR range (mm)	Ossification centres
2	69–80	11 pairs ribs: ilium: cervical neural arches: thoraco-lumbar vertebrae.
3	81–135	Sacral bodies: ischium: 2nd. phalanges hand.
4	136–175	Male pubis: male calcaneum.
5	176–215	Talus: female pubis and calcaneum: male sternal segments 1–3.
6	216–255	Sacral lateral masses.
7	256–285	All sternal segments: distal femur.
8	286–315	Cuboid: proximal tibia: humerus.

epiphyseal plane) may provide a misleading radiographic picture.' He further notes that Noback *et al.* (1960) have added to knowledge on this problem by reporting that from the beginning of *pre-fusion* (first radiological sign of epiphyseal union) to *fusion*, represented a time-elapse of 6·5–8·5 months. The mean of the pre-fusion period was 6·5±0·69 months, of the fusion period was 2·8±0·3 months for a 'fast' individual, 4·2±0·4 months for a 'slow' individual. The mean of the fusion process of a series of 15 hand epiphyses was 16 months (range of 4–28 months).

3 Radiology in forensic dentistry

The scope of medical forensic pathology is wide and the contribution of radiological techniques correspondingly diverse. In contrast, forensic dentistry as practised at the present time is concerned very largely with problems of identification. Assessment of facial injuries or comments upon the results of dental therapy may also find their way into the courts, but it is more usual in this country for the clinicians concerned with the assessment and treatment of such conditions to offer expert opinion should legal requirements make this necessary. It should not, however, be thought that the contribution of forensic dentistry is limited. Dentistry is no longer concerned solely with the study of the teeth and the immediately surrounding structures, but also with the whole of the craniofacial complex. For this reason dentists are experts on the growth and development of the skull and the contribution that this structure makes to facial characteristics used in identification.

The portrait artist or photographer makes use largely of the face and hands in presenting to his audience the identifying characteristics of the sitter, so it is perhaps not surprising that the most widely used method of identification of the dead is a visual examination of the facial features. Nuances of facial shape, contour, colour, muscle pattern, eye, nose and mouth characteristics along with hair pattern are imprinted in our minds. The extremely complex visual image of individuals whom we have known and a detailed analysis of the manner by which we recognize acquaintances has yet to be defined.

Returning to the cranio-facial complex, the situation

often arises when putrefaction of the soft tissues of the face or mutilation—intentional or otherwise—renders normal visual identification impossible or unacceptable to the next of kin (Fig. 3.1). Fortunately in these

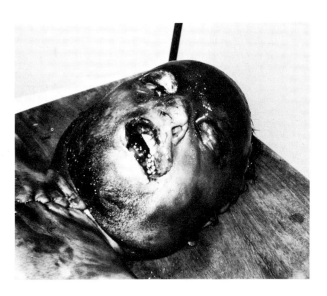

Fig. 3.1. The teeth are intact following extensive putrefaction.

circumstances the teeth, surrounding jaw bones and cranial bones are so complex that the means of identification may be present using a careful study of these characteristics. In addition, the cranio-facial structures have the advantage of being composed largely of hard tissues which are relatively indestructible. For instance, the enamel of human teeth constitutes by far the hardest tissue in the body and the teeth are protected to a large extent by the soft tissues of the cheeks and tongue which insulate them from traumas such as high-temperature fires, which would be expected to destroy most of the traditional identification features of the body. Not only are the teeth the most indestructible portion of the body, but their hard tissue portions develop over a long period of time extending from approximately 4 months after conception to 25 years of age. During this time they are subjected to all manner of environmental and systemic variations which may modify the growth of the teeth and may therefore be recorded within the structure of the tooth in a rather similar manner to the growth rings of a tree. Once built in to the teeth, information of this kind is permanently embodied because the hard tissues of the tooth are much less mobile than other tissues in the body.

The usefulness of the teeth in identification procedures resides not only in their resistance to damage but also in the fact that teeth are extremely complex and variable structures and vary between individuals in so far as shape, number, histological structure, arrangement within the jaws and so on are concerned. They are also routinely subjected in civilized communities to permanent alterations in structure brought about by the dental surgeon in his attempts to halt the ravages of dental decay. The mouth of a person who has received regular dental treatment is therefore a mine of information which is readily accessible either by direct observation or using radiographic techniques. This information may be used either to build up an individual 'identikit' picture of an unknown body or to provide data which can be compared with pre-existing records should a tentative identification be available.

In practice, the forensic dentist is usually faced either with an unknown body about which no information is available or he is requested to demonstrate that an unknown body is, or is not, that of a named individual for whom previous records are available. The former problem is by far the most difficult and may be referred to as identification by reconstruction. In such a reconstruction the forensic dentist seeks to deduce from the human remains available as much information as he is able. It may be possible under certain circumstances for the dental surgeon to give an opinion as to the age, the racial origin, the occupation or habits of the person involved, the sex, and various pointers as to the previous medical history. It will also be possible to provide a detailed description of the dental state of the individual in order that if records become available in the future a direct comparison may be made. This type of reconstructive activity will not in itself produce positive identification but may suggest possibilities or probabilities on which those investigating the case may build.

The second type of identification procedure may be

referred to as identification by comparison, and it is here that forensic dentistry comes into its own. Any previously charted information may be of use and will almost certainly include photographs of the deceased, particularly if the teeth are visible in a smile. Previous dental charts and records produced perhaps during a life-time of dental treatment may be supplemented by study models which may have been made of the mouth of the deceased in order that various oral appliances might be constructed. Interviews with the relatives of the deceased may lead to descriptions of dental appearances which can be compared with the situation in the unknown body. Photographs and study models constitute the most reliable evidence in comparison identification procedures since they are less subject to error or misinterpretation by the dentist or relative.

Also falling within this category are ante-mortem radiographs of the deceased which may have been taken during routine dental treatment. Dental radiography is now such a common procedure in dental surgery that almost every patient who has followed a course of treatment will have had one or more radiographs taken showing various features of the condition of the mouth. Such radiographs will demonstrate the details not only of the teeth but also of the surrounding bone and jaws and under certain circumstances radiographs may also have been taken of the cranio-facial structures. Considerable information may be derived from dental radiographs and may include not only the incidence of caries and periodontal bone loss of various types but also details of dental treatment ranging from simple filling procedures to complex specialized dentistry. Radiographs may reveal information not visible clinically, such as the presence of lining materials under fillings or the presence of materials used inside the teeth during root canal therapy. It may also be possible to detect previous oral surgery or prosthetic intervention in the form of implanted wires and plates related to jaw fractures or jaw remodelling procedures. The study of extraction sockets may contribute considerably to an understanding of the chronology of dental therapy which may have been carried out.

Other comparison identification techniques which have been used in the field of forensic dentistry include the correlation of radiographic images with photographs of the deceased in order to demonstrate, for instance, that a particular skull is that of a particular individual. In addition to reconstruction and comparison identifications, the problems of denture construction and type may yield considerable information which will be useful in identification procedures. A further aspect of forensic dentistry which is becoming increasingly important in criminal trials is the interpretation of bite marks produced at the time of an assault. The problem here is to determine whether a particular bite mark was inflicted by a particular individual.

This brief review of the scope of forensic dentistry would not be complete without mentioning the importance of microscopical techniques in relation to tooth and bone structure. The chemical and immunological study of samples of saliva and blood and the study of soft tissue features such as the shape of the palatal rugae and the presence of distinguishing intra-oral features such as pigmentation or the presence of chronic disease processes are also of considerable importance. Finally, the forensic dentist is frequently asked to comment upon fragments of dental tissues either at the scene of a crime or possibly in food-stuff materials, and radiography may play a part in the detection and identification of such items. Not all these aspects of forensic odontology make use of radiological methods but it is appropriate to review the specialized techniques of dental radiography in context, and in relation to the wider problems encountered in forensic dentistry. Details of the various techniques in which radiography is essential will be described in sequence.

IDENTIFICATION BY RECONSTRUCTION

Age estimation

It is not possible to estimate age accurately in every instance since there is considerable biological variation between individuals. Even if the techniques of age estimation were entirely satisfactory they would provide an indication of biological or dental age which may bear only a crude relationship to chronological age. Providing the forensic dentist is aware of this problem, however, and has carried out statistical evaluation of his techniques, he will be able to make a reasonably accurate estimate of age and be able to state the limits of accuracy of his estimation. Age determination from the teeth is not a new idea as it has been used for centuries by the horse-trading fraternity. Their techniques are based on the observation that horse incisors change their structural characteristics as they are worn down by the consumption of fibrous foods. The proportions and distribution of enamel and dentine on the worn biting surface of the teeth provide, therefore, a tolerable estimate of the age of the animal. In the human being, tooth wear of this degree is extremely rare in civilized communities, and although attrition does play a part in age estimation many other factors have also to be taken into account. Teeth develop initially as soft-tissue ingrowths from the oral mucosa. The tooth germs so produced go on to calcify, thereby becoming visible on radiographs. The crown of a tooth develops first and in the case of the permanent dentition crown formation may extend over a period of 3 or more years. At the completion of crown formation the root of the tooth commences to develop and this may take a further 3 or 4 years. During this period of root development the tooth begins to erupt into the oral cavity and eventually meets its antagonist in the opposite arch. From then on the tooth is subjected to wear and tear, the consequences of which can be expected to increase with age. All the techniques of age estimation from the teeth, therefore, are based upon examination of the state of calcification of the crown, the degree of development of the root and the eruption status or various subtle changes that occur within a tooth after it has reached its functional position. In so far as radiographic techniques are concerned it is the development of the teeth that is most important.

Development. The deciduous teeth commence calcification of the crowns at about 3–4 months after conception and the crowns continue to calcify beyond birth and into the neo-natal period (Fig. 3.2). The roots are usually complete between $1\frac{1}{2}$ and 3 years after birth. Commencement of calcification in the permanent teeth

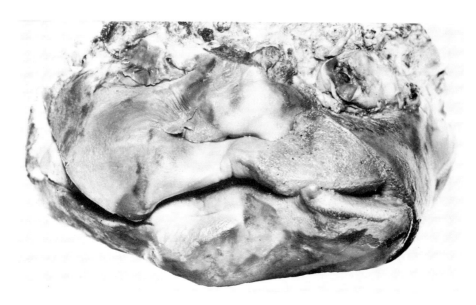

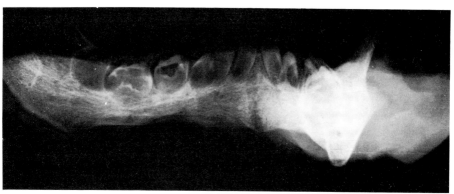

Fig. 3.2. (a) Putrefaction following burial. Age of a newborn child may be estimated from development of teeth. (b) Radiograph of mandible indicates dental development equivalent to 3 months of age (from Whittaker, 1977).

extends approximately over a 9-year period. The first permanent molar tooth begins to calcify at about birth whereas the third molar tooth, or wisdom tooth, does not commence hard tissue formation until 8–9 years of age.

The exact timing of calcification for an individual tooth can be quite variable. In the main, the data in the literature is based on charts prepared by Schour and

Fig. 3.3. Eruption sequence in man based on charts by Schour and Massler modified by Miles.

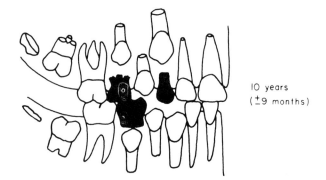

10 years
(±9 months)

Massler (1941) and Logan and Kronfeld (1933). (Fig. 3.3). Most workers have made use of data derived from these sources, but it has been recognized that because of the small sample sizes the range of variation may be much wider than these charts suggest. In addition Miles (1963) pointed out that the Schour and Massler chart does not record stages of growth of the third molar between 15 and 21 years. Its use is therefore limited to the lower age ranges.

For these reasons more recent studies of tooth development and eruption have been carried out, a very useful one being that by Moorrees *et al.* (1963). These authors studied 134 children by means of a longitudinal radiological study and presented in

Fig. 3.4. (a) Outlines of progressive stages of tooth development assessed from radiographs.

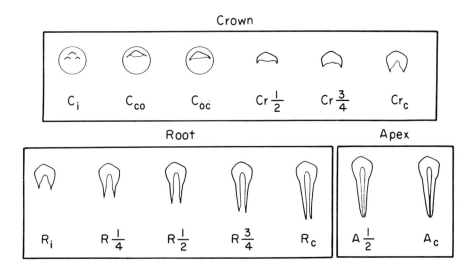

graphical form the mean age of crown, root and root apex development, along with standard deviations of the data. Both deciduous and permanent teeth were included in the survey and various stages of development were recorded in detail. An example of their method of presentation is shown in Fig. 3.4.

The limitations of the early tables and charts of tooth development were also recognized by Garn *et al.* (1959) who looked at three stages of formation of the mandibular pre-molar and molar teeth using serial oblique jaw radiographs. Their study included 255 white children from Ohio State, USA, and they used as their criteria the beginning of calcification in the crown, the

Fig. 3.4. (b) Chart illustrating tooth development at various ages for the upper and lower incisors (from Moorrees *et al.*, 1963).

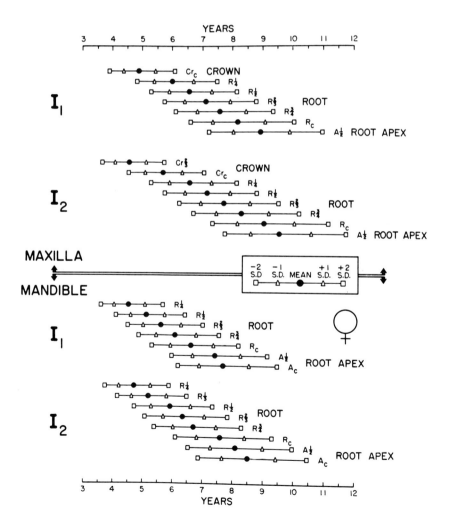

commencement of root formation and the final stage of apical closure of the root. They were able to show that teeth which develop later in the series were more variable than those at the beginning of the series; that the variability of development in males and females was about equal and that the actual ranges found were three times more than those which had been previously quoted.

A different approach to the problem was developed by Israel and Lewis (1971) who took as their standard the linear increase in tooth length as measured on standardized radiographs. They studied the lower left canine, pre-molars and second molar in 61 males and 65 females ranging in age from 6 to 34 years. Their technique was complicated, requiring specialized techniques of orientation, and is probably not easily applicable to the forensic situation.

Demirjian *et al.* (1973) proposed a new system in which each tooth is awarded a score according to which one of eight stages of development has been reached. The score is based on a total of 100 achieved by females of 16 years of age when the roots of the second molars are complete. Unfortunately, the system suffers from the same defect as the Schour and Massler chart in that the third molars are not included in their review. The system can consequently only be used in the younger age groups.

The third molar itself is a notoriously variable tooth in terms of development, but Miles (1963) concluded that although accuracy of age estimation decreases when using the third molar the error is not more than 2 years. Johanson (1971) studied third molar development radiologically and concluded that the use of this tooth can help to narrow the investigation to one age group of missing persons. Nolla (1958) has provided the most detailed description from radiographs of the developmental stages of the teeth. The degree of development of each tooth is awarded 1–10 points ranging from the time when no tooth crypt is present through the early stages of crown formation and ending in the closure of the root apex. Using the points awarded to each tooth, the age of the child can then be calculated by reference to tables of normal maturation in boys or in girls. The method does not appear to have been tested on a large scale and so the margin of error is not accurately known, but the data may nevertheless be extremely useful in conjunction with that produced by other authors.

A much simpler approach was that of Hunt and Gleiser (1955) in which age is estimated primarily from the degree of formation of the first permanent molar as seen on lateral jaw radiographs (see Fig 3.5). Miles (1958) tested the accuracy of this technique using radiographs of the mandibles of 58 children. He took into account the stage of development of the cheek teeth, and he was able to demonstrate that up to 12 years of age it is possible to estimate to within 18 months either way of the real age. From 12 years

Fig. 3.5. Radiographs of developing dentitions. (a) Age approximately $2\frac{1}{4}$ years. All the deciduous teeth are in occlusion. Permanent successors except second pre-molars are present. No evidence of tooth germ for second permanent molar. (b) Age approximately $8\frac{1}{2}$ years. Crown of second molar is complete. Apices of incisors and first molar incomplete.

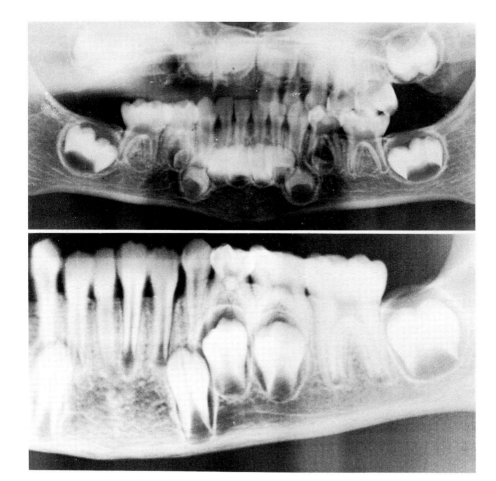

onwards, however, this becomes increasingly difficult and the estimated age departs from the real age on occasions by as much as 4 years.

It is clear, therefore, that there are many pitfalls in an accurate determination of age from radiographs of the teeth, but there is sufficient data available for a reasonably accurate determination to be made if all the available information is used. It is essential that high quality radiographs are available (Fig. 3.5) and it is also important that the sex is determined before the age estimation is carried out. It should also be remembered that certain pathological conditions may affect the growth and development of the teeth. It has been shown, however, by Sassouni that teeth are relatively less influenced by environmental forces in their formation and eruption than the growth of the skeleton. Shroff (1959) reported a case in which a mongol female was estimated to be 12–13 years of age from the skeletal remains, whereas the true age was finally established as 16 years.

Age from the facial skeleton. This problem has been dealt with in detail in the previous chapter, but is mentioned here briefly in relation to the paradental structures. Caffey (1950) surveyed the chronological history of the ossification and fusion of the sutures of the skull, but on the whole these are better examined by means of the naked eye rather than by means of radiographic techniques. It may be, however, that in certain specialized circumstances radiographs might be necessary to determine whether early closure of a suture has taken place.

Studies of the growth and development of the skull (Broadbent, 1937; Sassouni, 1960) have related facial size and proportions to age. Indeed this technique was used by the latter author in the identification of war dead. He commented that the range of variation was so wide that only approximate estimation of age could be achieved. Most of the data has been derived from studies of the developing facial complexes and therefore is inapplicable to age studies of the adult.

Race and sex determination

Race determination by direct examination of the skull is an extremely difficult procedure which should only be carried out by persons experienced in anthropological techniques. For this reason the place of radiography is extremely limited but certain features appearing on radiographs may, give a useful guide. It has been, for instance, suggested by Scott and Symons (1971) that the enamel of the molar teeth may extend down between the roots in Chinese races more commonly than in Europeans. The presence of enamel pearls on the roots of teeth may also be visible radiographically and this might indicate a person of Eskimo or Aboriginal origin. Congenital absence of the lower incisors is relatively rare but may be more common in Mongoloids (Lasker, 1950) and in natives of Malaya (Trotman, 1938). The pulp cavity in the molars of the Mongoloid race are said to be exceptionally deep and wide (Lasker & Lee, 1957), but apart from these examples information is meagre and racial determination from the teeth extremely difficult. The same problems apply to determination of sex and here it is useful to remember that the time of calcification of teeth is different in males and females (Nolla, 1958), but this in itself is of little use unless the skeletal remains can be aged by other means. In such cases early eruption of the teeth, particularly the mandibular canine (Hurme, 1957), would suggest the female sex rather than male.

The medical history

Indications that an individual has suffered from, or been treated for, certain diseases may be useful in the identification procedure. Many of the pathological processes affecting the skeleton will be reviewed in Chapter 4, but there are certain conditions associated with the teeth and jaws which are of particular interest to the forensic dentist. So far as the teeth themselves are concerned systemic diseases usually have to be present during the formative period to leave their mark. This is because the enamel and dentine are relatively stable once laid down and are not normally susceptible to disease processes occurring in other parts of the body. However, secondary dentine is being laid down throughout life and may therefore be susceptible to generalized disorders. The majority of these systemically produced defects in teeth are more easily seen clinically than radiologically, but certain ectodermal defects such as anhydrosis and ectodermal dysplasia may result in partial or complete anodontia which will require radiological examination for diagnosis. An increased incidence of supernumerary teeth is said to occur in persons with cleidocranial dysostosis and disturbed eruption patterns particularly of the permanent teeth may occur in both hyper and hypopituitarism. Other generalized conditions that are known to result in retarded eruption of the deciduous dentition are cretinism and rickets. In addition to changes occurring in the teeth there are a number of systemic disorders which may temporarily or permanently affect the jaws.

Certain systemic diseases produce radiolucent areas within the facial bones. These included Histiocytosis X, a term which covers eosinophilic granuloma of bone, Letterer–Siwe and Hand–Schüller–Christian syndrome.

In eosinophilic granuloma radiolucent areas of bone destruction, with sharply defined margins often attaining considerable size are characteristic features. As the lesions heal sclerosis develops around its borders.

Hand–Schüller–Christian disease is now regarded as the chronic form of Histiocytosis X. The skeletal lesions are very similar to eosinophilic granuloma but are usually more numerous. Lesions in the facial bones begin around the tooth roots but the teeth themselves are not affected.

Increased density of the facial bones may also be a manifestation of systemic disease e.g. osteopetrosis or Paget's disease. Bone absorption in the latter disease is the first manifestation followed by bone enlargement and sclerosis. Irregular dense sclerotic areas may form on the teeth. The maxilla is more often affected than the mandible.

Approximately 15% of all cases of monostotic fibrous

dysplasia and 20% of the polyostotic type have lesions in the jaws (Eversole *et al.*, 1972). The affected bones are expanded and show a homogeneous increase in density. The condition may affect the antrum, producing obliteration, and the orbital floor and zygomatic arch may also be affected. The lamina dura around the teeth and the space of the periodontal membrane can still be identified radiologically.

Although these systemic conditions will not enable a positive identification of an unknown body to be made they will add further information in a descriptive sense to the identikit picture of the individual concerned. Such information may enable hospital records to be traced and may at the very least enable some suspects to be eliminated from the enquiry.

In summary, reconstructive identification using radiographic techniques will not result in an immediate and positive identification but will provide information enabling a very detailed description of the unknown body to be made. It should certainly be possible up to the third decade to make a reasonable estimate of age from radiographs of the jaws alone and very much more accurate estimates may be made if teeth are sectioned and examined microscopically (Gustafson, 1950). It may prove possible to make some observations as to the likely sex and racial origin of the individual but from radiographs alone this is a much more difficult task. Finally the past medical or dental history as it affects the teeth or bones of the jaws may be permanently recorded and the results of such disease processes visible on radiographs. It would be a very unusual situation for the forensic dentist to have to provide information solely by the use of radiographs and they must be regarded therefore as providing supportive although very important evidence along with many other techniques available to the investigator.

IDENTIFICATION BY COMPARISON

Positive identification can only be achieved if antemortem records are available for comparison with the features of the unknown body. These ante-mortem records may include photographs of the individual, written dental records, study models or, ideally, radiographs. A great deal of information can be recorded in a single radiograph and it has been said (De-vore, 1977) that the single most accurate reliable source of information in an identification procedure is a comparison of ante-mortem and post-mortem X-rays.

The value of radiographs has also been emphasized by Stevens and Tarleton (1966) especially in relation to the mass disaster or air accident. Dental radiography is now such a routine procedure that most patients who have attended their dental surgeon on a regular basis could be expected to have had radiographs taken at some stage during their treatment procedures.

There have been some notable cases in the forensic literature where the presence of radiographs might have facilitated identification. Perhaps the most famous of these was the case of the charred corpses found outside Hitler's bunker as the Allies invaded Berlin. These bodies were identified by a dental technician but Furness (1976) regards it as the greatest omission in forensic science that skull and dental radiographs were not taken. This was a particularly serious omission since it is known that Hitler had skull radiographs taken in September 1944 following the unsuccessful attempt on his life (Fig. 3.6).

Another well-known case quoted by Saunders (1968) was the Moors murder case in which no ante-mortem dental records were available. The only specimen made available for examination by forensic dentists was the mandible of the girl and the most notable feature was the presence of a retained deciduous incisor on the left side. Radiological examination disclosed absence of the left first permanent incisor and both second premolars. These features would certainly have been sufficient for positive identification had ante-mortem radiographs been available. Dental radiographs may be used to look for peculiarities of anatomical form or of present pathology and they may also be important in determining therapy which has been carried out by the dental surgeon.

Fig. 3.6. Radiograph of Adolf Hitler following July bomb plot. Note complex and unique bridgework (from Sognnaes and Ström, 1973).

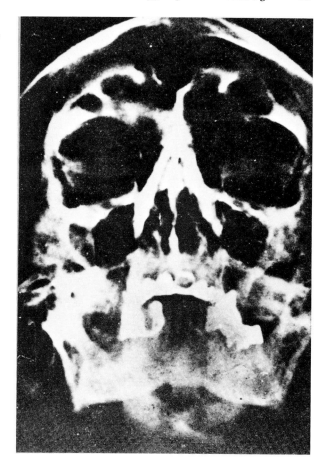

The teeth

The normal adult possesses 32 teeth and these are subject to variation in terms of shape, size, presence or absence and angulation within the jaws. Apart from the absence of teeth all these features are unfortunately subject to variation dependent upon the angulation of the X-ray beam at the time radiographs are taken. This problem will be dealt with in more detail when radiographic techniques are discussed.

Unless the occlusion is absolutely normal and is made up of the total number of teeth possible then radiographs may be of use in identification procedures even when no particularly unusual features are present. For instance it may be possible to show that an identification could not apply to an unknown body because ante-mortem radiographs reveal the absence of a particular tooth whereas the same tooth was present on post-mortem radiographs of the body (Fig. 3.7). The distribution of caries as seen on radiographs,

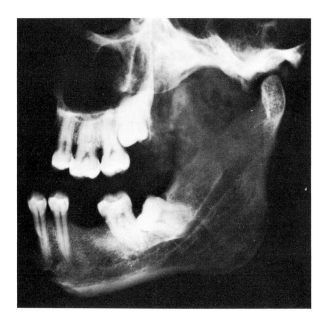

Fig. 3.7. Radiograph of fragment of dismembered body. Upper and lower wisdom teeth clearly visible and had been surgically removed from a person suspected of being same individual. Negative identification is therefore proved.

particularly bite wing radiographs, may be more or less unique to a particular person and may therefore be of some value in identification procedures. However, it must be remembered that caries is a progressive disease and therefore the pattern may differ markedly on X-rays taken post-mortem as compared to those taken ante-mortem. If a considerable time has elapsed between the two the presence of caries in the ante-mortem situation and its absence on a post-mortem radiograph would of course conclusively demonstrate that an error of identification had been made.

An interesting feature of the caries process is that it arrests at or shortly after death. The incidence of caries may therefore be determined in skeletal material and can be measured in ancient populations undergoing archaeological survey. This particular aspect of forensic dentistry will be dealt with in more detail below.

The other extremely common pathological condition

with which dentists have to deal is periodontal loss resulting in migration of the gingival attachment of the tooth towards the tooth apex, and more significantly to the radiologist, a loss of supporting bone around the tooth. This loss may be either horizontal so that all the teeth in an arch have suffered to more or less the same extent or it may be localized to individual surfaces of single teeth in which case vertical bone loss results. Because of the three-dimensional nature of the bone loss it is very difficult to compare two radiographs taken at different times unless great care is taken to ensure identical horizontal and vertical angulation of both the X-ray beam and the intraoral film. For this reason patterns of periodontal bone disposition are not particularly useful in forensic work.

It has been pointed out by Cameron and Sims (1973) that there may be some loss of detail in radiographs due to an increase in soft tissue thickness occasioned by the presence of gas from decomposition. The same authors have noted that teeth may loosen when such jaws dry out and in these cases the teeth should be pressed firmly back into the sockets in order that confusing variations in periodontal ligament thickness may not cause problems. Seward (1972) noted that tissues immersed in fixing solutions for a period of time tend to become somewhat more opaque than fresh tissues.

Anatomy of the skull

This aspect of comparative identification has been dealt with in more detail elsewhere but the forensic dentist must be aware of peculiarities of the supporting structures of the teeth since it may be necessary to comment on extra-oral jaw radiographs which are available for examination. Of all the bony structures of the cranium the air sinuses have been most often used in identification procedures. The first suggestion of their use appears to have been by Schuller (1921) and later by Culbert & Law (1927). They suggested the use of the nasal air sinuses in conjunction with radiographs of the mastoid air cells. Poole (1931) proposed a classification of the frontal air sinuses as seen on radiographs taking into account four criteria. These were the height and breadth and the presence or absence of the sinuses; the symmetry or otherwise and the deviation of the septum between the sinuses. The suggestion of such a classification seems never to have been followed up in detail although Schuller (1943) proposed a classification of the frontal air sinuses as radiographed in the forehead–nose position. This classification was somewhat more comprehensive and included the shape and deviation of the septum; the characteristics of the upper border; the presence or absence of the partial septum; any extensions into the ethmoid bone; the height from the planum and finally the breadth of the sinuses and the position of their mid line. Bostram *et al.* (1973) used the shapes of the frontal sinuses and the sellaturcica as identification features and Cheevers and Ascencio (1977) used the shape of the frontal sinuses in identification of a missing Canadian hunter. They commented that under normal circumstances the shape of the adult frontal sinus should remain unchanged throughout adult life and even identical twins have differing shapes of sinus. However, they do note that pathological changes such as Paget's disease, osteoma, osteosarcoma, or endo-cranial tumours may produce gross deformities in the sinus outlines.

Voluter (1959) believed the sellaturcica to be highly individualistic and also to be so protected as to be unlikely to be damaged by fire. However Thompson (1955) has pointed out that the shape of the sellatur-cica may change with age and also in the presence of tumours, acromegaly or Hand–Schüller–Christian's disease. Perhaps the most extensive use of skull radiographs in identification procedures was that by Sassouni (1960). He used lateral and postero–anterior radiographs taken on a cephalometer and eight measurements were taken from the postero–anterior films and eight from the lateral films. In the former instance the measurements were of the frontal sinus breadth, the facial height, the bigonial breadth, the cranial height from mastoid to apex, the incisor height, the bizygomatic breadth, the bimaxillary breadth and the maximum cranial breadth. In so far as the lateral films were concerned the eight measurements used were the height of the cranium, selected distances from the centre of the sellaturcica, the facial height and the cranial length as measured in selected positions. He carried out tests to see if identification from postero–anterior radiographs was possible in 498 cases. Using a computer into which the measurements were fed he demonstrated that it was possible to carry out direct identification in 97% of cases. The method appears to be promising but requires specialized expertise and in particular the availability of cephalometric X-rays taken ante-mortem. It would appear, however, that the technique could be adapted in order to produce standardized ante-mortem records of high risk personnel such as airline crews and the military.

Dental therapy

For the purposes of this discussion dental therapy may be divided into restorative procedures to replace either tooth tissue or missing teeth and secondly surgical procedures in which teeth or bony structures are excised or modified. Once a restoration is placed in a tooth it remains to all intents and purposes unchanged until it is either removed or lost. Exceptions to this general rule are the silicate cements, used for anterior restorations in former years, which have a high rate of solubility in saliva and also some of the lining materials placed under permanent restorations.

It has been reported recently (Akester, 1979) that lining materials of the calcium hydroxide type may become completely absorbed below amalgam restorations and comparison of ante-mortem and post-mortem radiographs in these circumstances may therefore be difficult. Many of the materials used to restore carious teeth are radio-opaque and are consequently demonstrated clearly on radiographs. The more complicated the shape of a restoration, the more useful it is in identification comparison procedures. Thus, amalgams with retaining pins placed into the dentine are often more useful than amalgams retained by conventional means but it must be remembered that in order to compare restorations of this type it is essential that post-mortem radiographs are obtained in an identical fashion to the ante-mortem radiograph.

More complex restorations such as gold bridges or fixed prostheses have been used in identification procedures even when the restoration has been found out of the mouth following, for instance, a hotel fire (Waaler, 1960). Although skull X-rays were not taken of the charred corpses found beside the Berlin bunker by the Russians and later identified as the bodies of Eva Braun and Adolf Hitler (Sognnaes & Strom, 1973) nevertheless the information derived from the ante-mortem radiographs of Hitler's skull taken at the time of the attempt on his life (September 1944) revealed several very characteristic dental restorations. These included a maxillary left central incisor with a metallic restoration of a window crown type and a special dental bridge in the right mandibular area with periodontal bone loss around the mandibular incisor roots. These features were compared with the various dental features described in the Russian autopsy report and in the opinion of the authors provide definite dental proof that the body autopsied by the Russians was that of Hitler (Fig. 3.6).

Although the crowns of the teeth and restorations present in them may be extremely useful in comparison exercises it is a fact that crowns become carious and restorations may become lost. The roots of the teeth are often more useful to the forensic dentist because apart from the possibility of caries attack from the crown, the roots tend to retain their shape and angulation since they are protected within the bone. The possibility of root resorption and drifting of teeth must, however, be borne in mind.

A classic case in which the roots of only a single tooth were present is that of the Dobkin murder of 1942 (Pedersen, 1965). A partially burnt dismembered body was found beneath a London church and radiographs of the maxilla revealed the presence of premolar roots. These post-mortem radiographs were compared with radiographs taken by a dental surgeon in 1934 when he extracted the premolar teeth leaving the fractured roots behind in the jaw bone.

Harvey (1976) comments that such conscientious preservation of radiographs by dental practitioners is unfortunately rare. Radiographs of tooth roots may be even more important, in the forensic sense, if root canal therapy has been carried out as the materials used in this procedure are radio-opaque and their position may be identified readily on radiographs. The adaptation of the root canal filling to the root canal is often quite characteristic so that a single radiograph of this type may be sufficient to enable a positive identification to be made (Fig. 3.8). It is beyond the scope of this book to attempt to categorize all the types of radio-opaque restorations which might be found in an individual but the examples given serve to indicate that the multiplicity of patterns produced on radiographs by the intervention of the dental surgeon whilst not being so individualistic as the fingerprint nevertheless help considerably in the identification of an unknown corpse.

Surgical intervention may also be recorded radiographically and may therefore be useful in identification procedures. The most common type of intervention is

Fig. 3.8. Ante- and post-mortem radiographs of air disaster victim. Characteristic shape of root, root filling and pulp chambers prove identification.

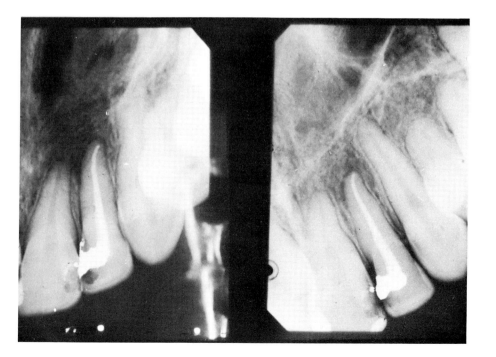

the extraction of teeth or roots of teeth and this in itself may provide useful information in that some estimation of the time since extraction may be gained by careful examination of a radiograph. After a tooth is removed the socket normally fills with blood and the clot eventually organizes resulting in resorption of the original socket wall, or lamina dura, and the filling of the socket area with new bone. It used to be thought (Leeuwen, 1948) that the time since extraction of the tooth could be accurately determined radiologically but it is now known that there are very considerable variations in the way sockets heal even in normal people. Occasionally sockets may be unchanged on radiographs up to 15 years after extraction of the tooth and even the lamina dura may be preserved during this time. Sometimes the lamina dura remains intact and sclerotic bone fills the socket giving the appearance of a retained root with a central root canal (Worth, 1963). As a general principle the timing of extraction socket healing should not be determined solely from radiographs but biopsies should be taken through the healing area. These have been shown to provide

Fig. 3.9. Dental burr left at site of operation results in positive identification.

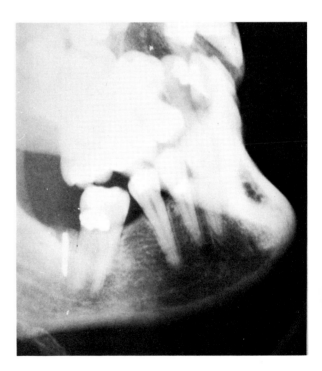

accurate estimations of the chronology of healing (Gustafson, 1966).

Valuable information regarding identification may result from dental surgery where accidental labelling of the site has occurred. Infrequently a radio-opaque steel burr may be left at the site of surgical removal of a tooth (Fig. 3.9) or radio-opaque amalgam may be lost from a tooth during extraction, fall into the blood filled socket, and become incorporated as a permanent marker in the bone. Events such as this will normally be fully recorded by the dental surgeon both in the form of ante-mortem radiographs and discussion in the patient's records and are often extremely useful when identification procedures become necessary.

If death occurs during protracted courses of oral surgical or prosthetic treatment the deceased may still harbour various devices in and around the mouth which are themselves indicative of specialized treatment. Circumferential bone wires are used in the treatment of fractures of the jaws and fragments of a bone in a convoluted fracture may be wired by open surgery. This type of treatment (Fig. 3.10) along with

Fig. 3.10. Results of treatment of fractured jaw help in identification procedures.

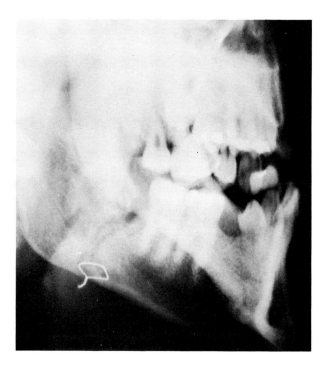

complex orthodontic treatment will again be carefully recorded during the treatment phase and ample records should be available for ante- and post-mortem comparison. The results of dental treatment may be demonstrable by the shape of edentulous jaws following the prescription of dentures. This may particularly be the case if pre-prosthetic surgery has been carried out and it may therefore sometimes be possible to determine whether or not an individual is likely to have worn dentures from certain features of the radiological appearance of the edentulous ridges. Interpretation of the radiographic appearance of the mouth after death is clearly a highly specialized procedure and comparison of post-mortem and ante-mortem radiographs whilst potentially yielding extremely useful information clearly requires the expert advice of the forensic dental surgeon.

Dental fragments

Occasions arise when small fragments of radio-opaque material become either impacted in soft tissues or are found at the scene of a crime or in foodstuffs. It may be necessary to determine whether these fragments are of dental origin. In most cases the fragment can be dissected out and investigated morphologically using a low-power dissecting microscopy and if dental tissues are present these may be recognized on ground section using light microscopic techniques (Yamamoto *et al.*, 1971). It has also been shown to be possible to determine the species of origin of small fragments of tooth using serological methods (Whittaker *et al.*, 1978). In some circumstances these techniques may not be applicable and radiography may then be the technique of choice.

Petersen and Kogan (1971) describe an air disaster in Canada in which 109 persons were killed and fragmentation of the bodies was considerable. These authors mainly used occlusal radiographs in order to produce data from the fragments which could then be compared with ante-mortem records. 60% of all the identifications were aided by dental evidence and the authors make the point that if on-the-spot radiographic facilities had been available it would have been possible to locate many more dental fragments. Not only is radiography of vital importance in determining the shape and character of buried fragments but it may also be the only means of initially locating such fragments. For these reasons it has been suggested that radiography of the head and neck in cases of gross fragmentation should be carried out routinely. On occasions, for example following severe fires, it may be difficult or impossible to determine whether small fragments collected at the scene of the incident are in fact bone or tooth fragments or simply fragments of debris. Johanson (1960) described a technique for establishing from dental fragments how many individuals have been involved in a catastrophe. The method has since been improved (Johanson & Saldeen, 1969) and now involves X-ray transparent plastic boxes in which debris can be collected and fragments such as teeth, dental restorations or bullets can be easily located. In a case described by Gustafson (1966) only a handful of bone, teeth and dental restorations in the form of fillings and a bridge could be found following a house fire. From these and from radiographs of them it was possible to fit the pieces of teeth together and produce a positive identification.

When fragments of teeth are collected some weeks or months after loss from the host animal it may prove impossible to determine the species of origin using serological techniques (Whittaker *et al.*, 1979). In such instances radiographs of the tooth fragment would be useful in determining the origin. A fragment of a tooth (Fig. 3.11) was found in a sandwich sold in a restaurant. Radiological examination of the fragment revealed an unusual pulp and root canal morphology which was eventually matched to that of the 2nd premolar of the domestic pig. Radiographs were taken of a pigskull using similar angulation and it can be seen that the outline of the fragment is that of a portion of the premolar pig tooth.

Radiographs are, of course, of particular value where it is suspected that a tooth fragment lies embedded in soft tissues (Fig. 3.12).

Fig. 3.11. (a) Radiograph of tooth fragment. (b) Radiograph of pigs premolar. The fragment is identifiable as the distal root of this tooth.

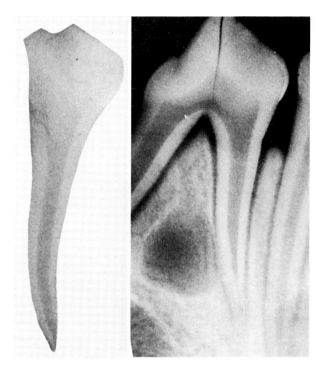

Fig. 3.12. Tooth fragment embedded in lip following trauma.

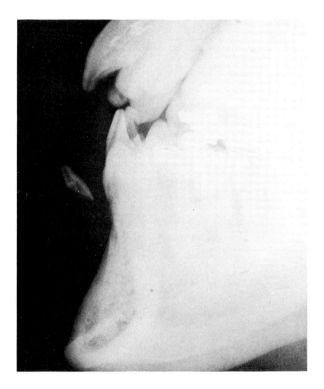

Reconstruction from radiographs and ante-mortem photographs

There are very few cases in the forensic dental literature in which use has been made of superimposition techniques involving ante-mortem photographs and post-mortem radiographs. The classic case in which this technique was developed was that of the murder of his wife and maid by Dr Ruxton in September 1935. Dismembered remains were found of the two women and Glaister and Brash (1937) used scale photographs of Mrs Ruxton and her maid and superimposed these upon radiographs of the skulls in which care was taken to angle the remains in exactly the same manner as was present in the photographs. Although this particular evidence was not used in the trial it nevertheless remains a classical account of the problems and solutions involved in techniques of this nature. A similar technique was used by Furness (1976) in which superimposition of a photograph of the teeth and face onto a photograph of the teeth and skull gave 23 points of comparison, resulting in a positive identification. In this particular case radiographs of the skull were not used. It has been suggested by Furuhata and Yamamoto (1967) that using radiographs only, facial features may be reconstructed on a skull by employing average tissue thicknesses at various reference points. Glaister and Brash (1937) felt that reconstruction of soft tissue features in this way from radiographs were not satisfactory but the technique is still under investigation in several centres.

RADIOGRAPHIC TECHNIQUE

It is outside the scope of this book to describe in detail all the available techniques of dental radiography. These may be found in the standard texts on the subject. Forensic dentists may make use of the standard intra-oral and bite wing radiographs, occlusal intra-oral radiographs, lateral obliques and anteroposterior radiographs and also orthopantomographs. It may also be necessary on occasions to employ special techniques to demonstrate the paranasal air sinuses or other specific features. In general it is important to select tube and film angulations which will result in the minimum of distortion of the particular structure to be radiographed. In comparisons of ante-mortem and post-mortem radiographs, the ante-mortem radiographs should be, if possible, available at the time the post-mortem radiographs are produced in order that comparable views may be taken. The logistical problems of acquiring post-mortem radiographs are often considerable. Although the normal dental X-ray machine is suitable for producing intra-oral radiographs and the simpler extra-oral views, and its use is familiar to all dental surgeons, it nevertheless has its limitations and indeed may not be available either in the mortuary or out in the field.

Because of the decomposed and unpleasant nature of many of the specimens requiring identification it is often not appropriate to transfer them to a hospital department of radiology where there may be problems keeping the material separated from the normal patient through-put and the radiologist may not be experi-

Fig. 3.13. Method of supporting skull on polystyrene block for orthopantomogram.

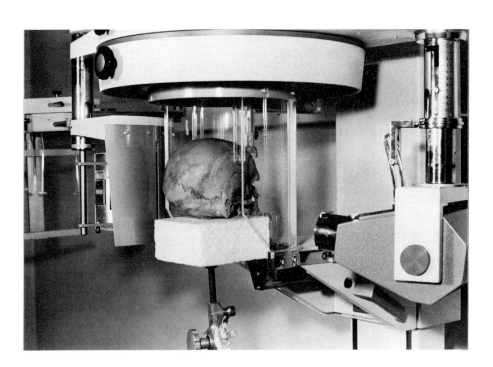

enced in dealing with this type of material. For these reasons it is often preferable to remove the maxilla and mandible from the corpse having gained the coroner's permission so to do. These fragments may then be carefully examined in the laboratory under ideal conditions of lighting and may then if necessary be preserved before radiographs are taken. Although in theory it is better to use a non-destructive technique like radiography of the intact body if facilities are available, the recommended course of removal of segments of the jaws, whilst being a second best, may well result in much better radiographs, the quality of which may out weigh the disadvantages. (Figs. 3.13 and 3.14).

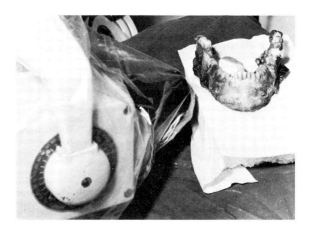

Fig. 3.14. Use of intra-oral film held in place by plasticine. Note covering of machine to avoid contamination.

Processing techniques

Ante-mortem radiographs to be used for forensic purposes must be of high quality and must be fixed satisfactorily in order to retain detail. Radiographs where fixation has been poor may be improved by re-washing and re-fixing at the time of examination. Even when old, badly exposed or developed, or otherwise unsatisfactory films are all that is available it will still be of importance to gain as much information as possible from them. A technique for improving detail from seemingly useless radiographs has been described by Sparks (1973) in which copies are made with a light

path travelling twice through the photographic emul-
sion being copied so that contrast and details are
improved.

It may on occasion be necessary for duplicates to be
produced of radiographs to be used in evidence. On the
whole duplicates should not be used for court evidence
but only retained by the forensic dentist as second
copies. Satisfactory copies may be made on Kodak
radiographic duplicating film by means of contact
printing, or 35 mm slide copies may be made using a
high quality black and white reversal film. It must be
remembered that duplicates are rarely as good as the
original.

Marking and mounting

It is essential that any radiographs taken specifically for
forensic purposes must be clearly marked at the time
the radiograph is taken in order that continuity of
evidence may be preserved. Any comparison of anti-
and post-mortem dental radiographs is totally dependent upon the correct identification of the radiograph
itself. A simple way to carry out this labelling (Kogon &
Reid, 1974) is to place a small piece of lead foil sheet
from a dental film packet on the tube side of an exposed
film packet in an area outside the picture field. A
suitable code may be marked on the lead foil sheet
using either a ball-point pen or a typewriter without
ribbon. After exposure the code appears on the film.

The mounting and viewing of radiographs may also
present problems in the forensic dental field. It is usual
for various technical reasons to examine and evaluate
radiographs from a position behind the film, that is, to
view through the X-ray film towards the X-ray tube.
Dental radiography however, used techniques which
may make this viewing method difficult.

Because of ready access to the oral cavity intra-oral
positioning of X-ray films is common practice in the
dental field and has the advantage of bringing the
object to be radiographed, for example the tooth, close
to the film. These intra-oral films are necessarily small
and therefore full mouth radiography requires between

10 and 14 separate exposures. For ease of viewing, these films are normally mounted using the Zigmondy tooth classification system (Fig. 3.15). For these reasons the International Dental Federation (FDI) now recommend that intra-oral radiographs should be mounted as seen from the tube side. They also recommend that films taken at the same visit should all be mounted together and marked not only with the name of the patient but also with the name of the dental surgeon.

Fig. 3.15. Maxillary intra-oral radiographs mounted in sequence. Upper left quadrant is designated by number 2 followed by the number of the tooth in the permanent dentition.

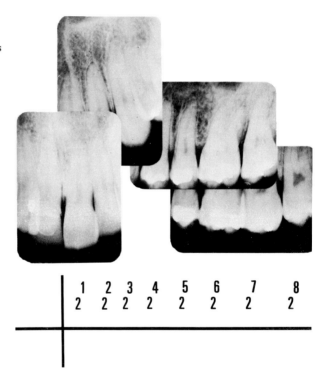

1	2	3	4	5	6	7	8
2	2	2	2	2	2	2	2

DENTAL RADIOLOGY IN ARCHAEOLOGY

Although at first sight archaeology would seem to be a far cry from forensic dentistry in fact they are more closely related than one might suppose. Skeletal remains may be discovered and reported to the police whose interest is one of determining whether a crime has been committed or the remains are of recent origin requiring identification. Under these circumstances it may be possible for the forensic dentist to conclude whether the remains are ancient and of no direct interest to the law enforcement agencies. As described earlier in this chapter, one aspect of forensic dentistry is concerned with a detailed description of an unknown body. The techniques that are available may equally well be applied to the study of anthropological or archaeological material, and indeed have been so applied in the past. Most of the studies on archaeological material have been concerned with estimates of caries incidence (Moore & Corbett, 1971) and in the problems of age determination, largely from eruption sequence and attrition patterns of the teeth (Miles, 1958). Radiographs may be useful in the assessment of large populations of skeletal material although they appear to have been infrequently used on a routine basis. In the younger age groups they can, as previously described, result in a more accurate age estimate using the degree of development of the tooth crowns rather than the eruption status (Fig. 3.16). In addition they may be useful in determining whether

Fig. 3.16. Romano-British mandible showing developing permanent premolar and second molar. Age is estimated at approx. $8\frac{1}{2}$ years.

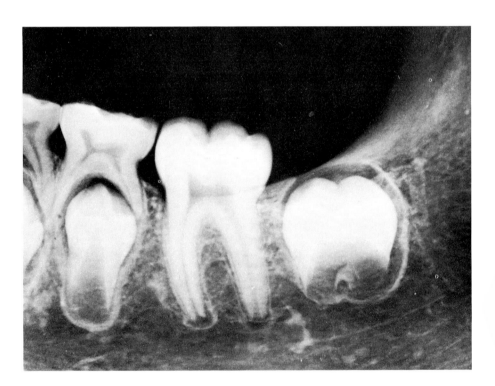

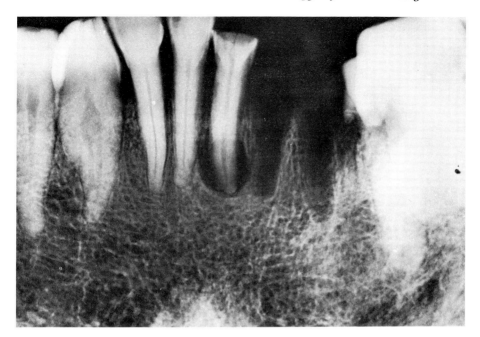

Fig. 3.17. Radiolucent area at apex of central incisor indicates ante-mortem damage to this tooth.

lesions of the tooth crowns are due to ante-mortem caries or to post-mortem soil damage. Apical changes in the surrounding bone would of course confirm the former (Fig. 3.17). Estimates of caries in archaeological material are based on the numbers of decayed and missing teeth per mouth and it is consequently important to make some estimate of whether any missing teeth were lost before death (due to caries or periodontal loss) or after death. If this is not done, the total caries experience may be artificially depressed and the extent to which this has occurred would be unknown. Radiological examination of the tooth sockets can help in this problem.

Radiographic techniques have on occasions provided interesting information for the historian. In 1912 a Mr C. Dawson found a fossil skull of 'Piltown man'. In all, between 1911 and 1913, four pieces of cranium, a jaw, nine remnants of animal teeth, 5 flints and a canine tooth had been discovered. Finally in 1915 Dawson found the remains of yet another individual 2 miles away. The second Piltdown man was the last of the sensational discoveries. Further discoveries in the 1930s of Java man and of Australopithicus in the eastern rift valleys of Africa indicated that man appeared to have evolved in a different manner to that indicated by Piltdown. In 1955 after some years of study it was proved that the Piltdown fragments were a hoax and that the fluorine content of both jaw and cranium were markedly different and indicated an age of no more than 50 000 years (Oakley & Weiner, 1955). What has become the most celebrated forgery in the whole of science was in part exposed because dental radiographs showed that the teeth had been ground down artificially. A cuspid tooth, one of the key pieces of evidence in the original find, was also shown by radiographs to have been ground down and the root canal filled with grains of a mineral mixed with a cement-like substance.

Moving onwards in the development of the civilization of man, the radiological aspects of forensic dentistry have played their part in the investigation of an era when man preserved his remains in anticipation of the after life. Radiographs were taken of some of the Egyptian Royal Pharoahs when they were first discovered but with the advent of more sophisticated equipment new information has come to light. Harris *et al.* (1966) described a portable cephalometer with a radioactive X-ray source of Ytterbium 169 so that no external power source was required. They used polaroid X-ray film in order to carry out cephalometric surveys in Nubian cemeteries. This followed their extensive studies of the royal Pharoahs in the museum in Cairo using standard radiographic equipment in which they were able not only to describe the caries incidence and periodontal status of these individuals but also to demonstrate family similarities in cranial and dental relationships in some of the Pharoahs examined. Radiographic techniques were attempted on the examination of the Tutankhamun mummy (Leek, 1971) and in this instance a radioactive source contained within a hypodermic needle was inserted through the cheek into the oral cavity resulting in acceptable extra-oral radiographs.

Rushton (1965) reported on his examination of a fifteenth-century child skeleton said to be that of Lady Ann Moubray, the child bride of Richard, one of the Princes in the Tower. From historical records she was believed to have died at the age of 8 years 11 months in 1481 and Rushton was able to demonstrate from the dental radiographs that the age at death was approximately correct. He also noted that the upper and lower left second permanent molars were absent from the skeleton and this is of some interest since Tanner and Wright (1935) demonstrated congenitally missing teeth in the Princes in the tower especially in the jaws of Edward V. This may have been a familial trait since Ann Moubray in addition to being married to Richard was also closely related to the Princes.

An unusual skull was that examined by Renson (1970) in that it had been recovered from beneath the sea off the Isle of Scilly at the site where in 1707 a number of ships had foundered in a storm, one of these being the Flagship HMS 'Association'. Using radiographic techniques he was able to demonstrate that there was no secondary dentine in the pulp chambers of the teeth and the spheno-occipital synchondrosis was still unclosed. He aged the skull at approximately 15 years at the time of death.

An extensive survey on more recent material was carried out by Shuff (1976) on 66 nineteenth-century skulls. Cephalometric tracings of lateral skull radiographs were made and it was demonstrated that there was a deficiency in forward growth of the mandible possibly due to malnutrition and an increase in the angle formed by the mandibular and SN planes also probably due to malnutrition. Shuff also demonstrated that when radiographs alone were used to estimate the age of subjects who were less than 20 years of age the mean error was approximately one year.

In 1517 the Spaniards invaded Mexico and discovered on the Yucatan Penninsula a highly advanced civilization. Amongst many other social and religious practices the Maya had developed a sophisticated technique for the placement of gold inlays in the labial surface of the anterior teeth. For many years there was doubt as to whether these inlay cavities were prepared ante- or post-mortem but radiographs reported by Fastlicht (1948) clearly demonstrated that there were pulpal changes occurring after the inlay cavities had been prepared. In this case therefore radiographs have added considerably to our knowledge of the techniques employed by these fascinating peoples.

In addition to the study of human archaeological remains, dental radiography has been employed in the study of archaeological artefacts. Near-Eastern cylinder seals were studied by Gorelick (1975) using a dental machine operating at 90kV and 15mA. It had previously been suggested that seals which were copies of originals would possess a straight centre hole whereas the original cylinders would possess a crooked centre hole since they were drilled from both ends. He found in fact that he was unable to differentiate between the originals and copies using this type of techniques. The type of stone used in the construction of seals and the methods employed by the manufacturers were demonstrated by the radiographs.

THE LEGAL POSITION

In the early days of dental radiography, radiographs were not acceptable in courts of law as evidence. However, Sweet (1938) records that at that time they were fully acceptable in an American court of law and considered that 'one picture was worth a thousand words'. He was of the opinion that a jury was able to understand a radiograph when explained to them more readily than they would comprehend dental terminology. It is of course essential that whenever radiographs are produced as evidence they must be the originals and they must have been identified by an efficient marking method. A suitable technique has been described previously and the simple method of writing a coded number on the film using pencil in the dark room was reported by Harvey (1946). In order that ante-mortem radiographs be available for comparison techniques in forensic dentistry it is necessary that practitioners not only label their X-rays efficiently but also catalogue them with the patients' records. It also goes without saying that records must be kept for a reasonable length of time after treatment is complete. In Scotland the law demands that medical records must be kept for four years after the patient has ceased to be treated. It appears that in England and Wales the legal limit is as low as 18 months (Harvey, 1975). The defence societies in England and Wales recommend that medical records should be kept at least six years. The terms and conditions of service of dental practitioners working within the health service in England rule that all radiographs taken or obtained by the dentist as part of treatment must be retained for a period of 12 months after completion of that treatment. It seems clear that from a forensic point of view the recommended time scales are woefully inadequate.

Ownership of dental radiographs within the British general dental practitioner services is vested in the dentist himself. However, he is required to keep such records, including radiographs for the periods mentioned above, and during this time will produce records to the dental estimates board if so required. In the case of radiographs produced in hospitals within the National Health Service the radiographs would remain the property of the Area Health Authority within whose area the radiographs were taken. Permission must be sought therefore by the forensic dentist for removal and use of such records for legal proceedings.

SUMMARY

Radiological techniques now form an indispensable part of the science of forensic dentistry and are invaluable when reconstructive techniques have to be used in order to describe in detail the features of an unknown body. They are of even more importance when a comparison with ante-mortem radiographs is possible. The forensic dentist may be able to pronounce upon the likely age, sex and race of origin of the individual and may be able to contribute towards an understanding of the medical history. When comparison techniques are used the unique characteristics of the teeth themselves, therapy which they have been subjected to, and the treatment of conditions in the surrounding tissues may all provide useful identification features. Standard techniques of dental radiography are all that are necessary in the forensic field but they may require modification depending upon the particular situation. It is very important that special precautions be taken to continue the chain of evidence through from the specimens removed at post-mortem to radiographs finally produced, as evidence. If these safeguards are routinely taken, the combination of radiographic and dental techniques provide a significant contribution to forensic medicine as a whole.

The need to take adequate pre- and post-operative radiographs in the course of many dental procedures can not be over-emphasized as being an essential part of good clinical practice. Additionally they may provide vital evidence to enable a practitioner to defeat successfully an allegation of negligent treatment and in this context the availability of adequate radiographs is particularly important in the following instances:

(a) To determine the presence, position and form of unerupted teeth before deciding on extraction for orthodontic treatment.
(b) Prior to extraction of impacted, misplaced, fractured or clinically abnormal teeth.
(c) For the assessment of bone loss prior to treatment for periodontal disease.
(d) To determine the viability of teeth to be used as bridge abutments.
(e) To determine the presence or absence of retained roots before the construction of a bridge and possibly before the provision of dentures where there has been a history of difficult extractions.
(f) In endodontic treatment.
(g) In assessment prior to implant treatment.
(h) To check for interstitial caries.
(i) Where a fracture of the jaw is suspected.

Radiographs must, of course, be of adequate quality and reasons for obtaining poor films include incorrect angulation of the tube, incorrect exposure, movement of the patient, and incorrect developing technique. If the radiographs are in any way unsatisfactory, they should be retaken and, of course, checked to ensure that they contain the total information required.

For example, the radiograph of a patient with an impacted third lower molar should demonstrate:

(a) the whole tooth to be removed.
(b) the adjacent hard tissue.
(c) the relationship of the apices to the inferior dental neuro-vascular bundle.
(d) the relationship of the apices to the lower border of the mandible.

The value of occlusal and extra-oral radiography should not be forgotten although the latter is becoming more commonplace with the wider use of sophisticated pan-oral type apparatus. Even the usually excellent radiographs produced by such machines, have limitations and the use of good intra-oral bite wings in detecting early interstitial caries is still unsurpassed.

The defence organizations frequently receive requests for assistance from members against whom allegations of negligence are made following the provision of endodontic treatment, during the course of which a root canal reamer or broach is fractured and retained, and also when a root is unknowingly perforated. If a post-operation radiograph is not taken the opportunity to detect a small portion of an instrument that has fractured, or any other untoward occurrence, is missed. Such an allegation is often made after the patient complaining of pain from a recently root-filled tooth, has visited another practitioner, who will almost certainly take a radiograph, thereby bringing the mishap to the patient's attention. Had the first practitioner taken a radiograph and diagnosed the complication of treatment, and given an appropriate explanation to the patient, the likelihood of a claim for compensation would have been significantly reduced.

Radiographs are considered to be an integral part of the patient's dental records and not the property of the patient even though he may have paid for them. Should a patient transfer to another dentist there can be no objection to the complete dental records, either originals or copies, being sent to the new practitioner. They should, however, be sent directly to him and not given to the patient.

Negligence may not necessarily be proven because a practitioner has failed in a certain instance to take an X-ray film. However the law demands that a practitioner shall at all times exercise reasonable skill and care and in some cases this may well require radiographs in addition to visual and clinical examination. Difficulty will be experienced in defending a dentist who has extracted teeth for orthodontic purposes only to find later that certain teeth he believed would subsequently erupt were either congenitally absent or in such a position as to preclude any possibility of normal eruption.

Modern teaching impresses upon students that partially erupted wisdom teeth should be X-rayed prior to extraction and failure to do this followed by a fracture of the jaw during extraction may well constitute negligence. Similarly, a fracture occurring when an X-ray film gives inadequate coverage may lead to an allegation of negligence.

The provision of dentures for a patient giving a history of difficult extractions is unwise without previous radiological examination to exclude the possibility of retained roots, as also is the provision or attempted provision of root canal therapy, post crowns, bridgework, etc., without similar precautions. It must also be realized that negligence may be alleged if X-ray films are incorrectly taken or processed and thus prove of little diagnostic value; finally failure to note the presence or absence of a particular item on an X-ray film may be construed as negligence.

4 Radiology in forensic pathology

The largest single topic in the application of radiology to problems in forensic pathology is undoubtedly in identification, but as this has been fully dealt with in previous chapters, the present discussion will concern a number of other areas in which radiology can be of considerable or vital assistance to the forensic pathologist.

Gunshot wounds

In both the living and the dead the use of radiology is of prime importance in the investigation of firearm wounds. Naturally, where the victim is still alive, radiology plays a major role in treatment, localizing the projectiles and fragments and identifying damaged organs prior to surgical intervention. Such clinical radiographs may later be of evidential value if criminal proceedings arise from the events which led to the gunshot wound.

The most common medico-legal use of radiology in firearm wounds is as an adjunct to autopsy. Every experienced forensic pathologist is well aware that the retrieval of bullets, shot and fragments from a wound may be an extremely difficult, tedious and sometimes unrewarding task. Without the benefit of radiology, the search for such metallic fragments may be prolonged and untoward damage may be done to the tissues, perhaps leading to a reduction in the value of other pathological evidence.

Not infrequently, the projectile or projectiles take such an erratic course through the body that mere dissection fails to reveal the missile. It is one of the prime objects of an autopsy on the victim of a fatal gunshot wound to retrieve the missile in an intact and unmarked condition, so that it may be used by the forensic science laboratory in the tracing of the culprit weapon. In the case of rifled weapons such as pistols and rifles, the internal spiral machining of the barrel marks the projectile in a manner unique to every weapon, so that test-firing from a suspect weapon may produce a matching bullet with identical grooving from the rifling marks. For this technique to be successful, the bullet from a victim must be recovered without damage. Extensive blind dissection may hamper or even ruin this matching, as if the bullet is unexpectedly encountered with a sharp scalpel or forceps, the delicate markings may be scarred and partly obliterated, especially if a soft missile such as a lead revolver bullet is involved.

Radiology, by pinpointing the position of the projectile before dissection starts, is of great assistance in obviating this risk. In addition, the actual location of the missile or missiles can be accurately determined prior to dissection, thus saving time, effort and tissue damage.

On occasions, the missile may lodge in a most unpredictable site, quite remote from the entrance wound. Without radiology it might be almost impossible to discover it, without lengthy and perhaps disfiguring dissection. As an example, in a notorious gang-land murder some years ago, the victim was shot with a revolver, one entrance wound being in the upper chest near the shoulder. The autopsy was commenced without radiological facilities and no bullet corresponding to this wound could be found in the thorax or abdomen. The autopsy had to be suspended and the body removed to a hospital mortuary, where radiological facilities were available. It was then found that the projectile was adjacent to the hip joint, having tracked through the tissues in the most unexpected manner. Without radiology, it would have been extremely difficult to have retrieved the missile and certainly an untoward delay would have occurred in the investigation of the homicide.

Apart from the actual retrieval of missiles, radiology may be useful in determining the exact course of a missile through the body and hence assist in reconstructing the circumstances of the fatal discharge. Though as has been said above, the course of the bullet may be extremely erratic—usually due to deflection by bony structures—in most instances the final lodgement of the missile is at the end of a straight track from the entrance wound, if contact with solid objects such as bone or perhaps liver can be excluded. Thus a line from this point on the X-ray film to the entrance wound can be projected outside the body to give the direction of the trajectory and where films in different planes are employed, this can be evaluated on a three-dimensional basis.

However, a note of caution must be introduced here, as there is a danger of over-interpretation. This is due to the fact that although radiology may assist other methods in determining the trajectory *relative to the body*, it is naturally unsafe to relate this absolutely to external landmarks, as the body may not be in the erect or otherwise expected posture when struck by the bullet. A calculation of the path of the missile within the body cannot necessarily be used to determine the direction of approach unless good collateral evidence is available of the posture of the body at the time—evidence which is rarely offered.

Where shotguns are employed, the general spread of pellets can be determined and again an estimate made of the direction between the centre of the shot grouping so that the projection can be made from there through the entrance wound to give the line of fire. The size of the dispersion pattern of shot may also assist in an estimate of the distance of discharge, as the dispersion pattern from a shotgun consists of a long, narrow cone.

Where a single projectile is involved, there is often a difference in the appearances of the wound both anatomically and radiologically, depending upon the velocity of the missile. Revolvers may have a relatively low muzzle velocity of around 500 ft per second, whereas a military rifle may have a muzzle velocity of several thousand feet per second. As the mass of a bullet is relatively small, velocity is of great importance in contributing to the energy of an impact, and hence the amount of tissue damage and penetration.

When a low velocity missile traverses the head, the bullet may remain within the skull vault and be rendered visible on radiology. Even small ·177 air rifle pellets may penetrate the skull of a child and traverse the vault, though it never produces an exit wound. On the other hand a high velocity injury always produces an exit wound, often extremely disruptive in nature due to the transfer of energy to bone and other tissues. The track of a missile through soft tissue causes lateral transferred energy with cavitation into which the adjacent tissue oscillates violently within the space of a few milliseconds. Thus the track may be several times wider than the actual missile and sometimes air is found in this track, having been sucked into the wound behind the missile. Fragments of bullet and bone may also be seen along the missile track on radiology.

An example of a high velocity injury is shown in Fig. 4.1(a–b). An entrance wound was present in front of the right ear below the zygomatic arch and there was an exit wound behind the right ear. Fragments of bone are shown displaced into the brain to a depth of approximately 4·5 cm. Extensive fractures in the vault are shown in Fig. 4.2, following a tangential missile injury to the vertex. The air mentioned above can be seen in Fig. 4.3.

In low velocity missile injuries, the bullet is frequently found in the skull as mentioned earlier (Fig. 4.4(a–b)). A complete quadraplegia in another case resulted from a gunshot wound entering the left cheek, shattering the mandible and the bodies of C4 and C5. A large pre-vertebral haematoma was present in the cervical region. Myelography showed swelling of the cord with obstruction at the level of C6 (Fig. 4.5(a–b)).

Bony damage can also be estimated readily on radiography. When either a shotgun discharge from a smooth bore weapon or a single projectile from a rifled weapon is present, the impact of such projectiles against bone may cause secondary fragmentation and severe secondary tissue damage from the transfer of

Fig. 4.1. (a and b). Fragments of bone displaced deep into the brain tissue. An accidental discharge of a machine gun produced an entrance wound in front of the right ear and an exit wound behind the ear.

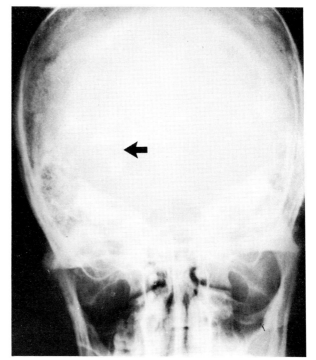

(a)

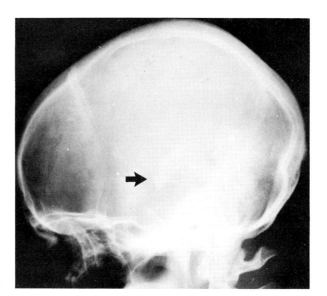

(b)

Fig. 4.2. High velocity tangential missile injury to the vertex of the skull producing extensive fractures.

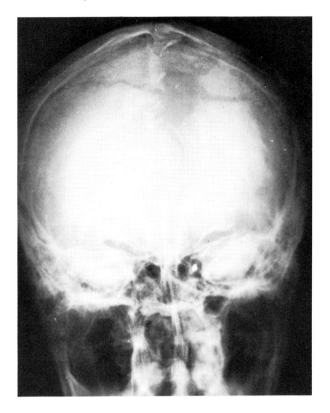

Fig. 4.3. High velocity missile injury with the entry wound in the occipital region close to the mid-line. Air was sucked into the wound behind the missile and is shown in the missile track posteriorly and also in the anterior horn of the lateral ventricle close to the bullet.

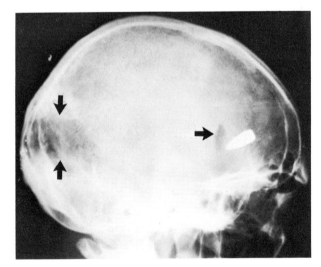

Fig. 4.4. (a and b). Low velocity missile injury with a fracture of the left frontal bone and the bullet lodged in the posterior parietal region.

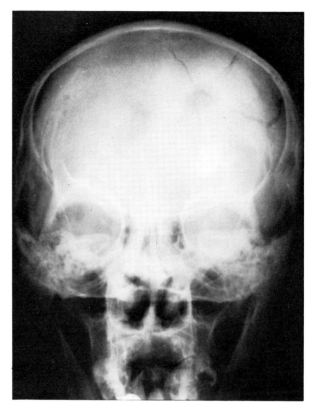

(a)

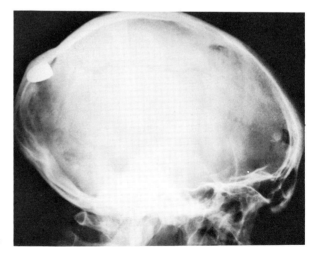

(b)

Fig. 4.5. (a and b). Low velocity gun-shot wound the bullet fracturing the bodies of the 4th and 5th cervical vertebrae. A large pre-vertebral haematoma is shown.

Clinically there was a complete quadriplegia and myelography showed obstruction to the flow of myodil with swelling of the cord.

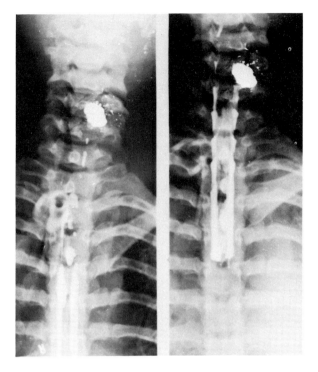

(a)

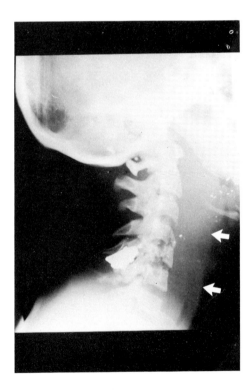

(b)

Fig. 4.6. Exit wounds in the back of the neck produced by sharp fragments of cervical vertebrae. (From Tedeschi C. Eckert W. & Tedeschi L. (1977) *Forensic Medicine.* W. B. Saunders, Philadelphia.

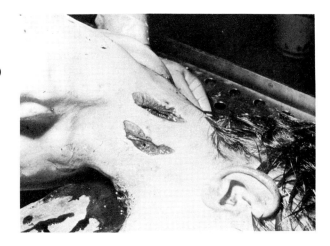

Fig. 4.7. Gun-shot wound producing extensive soft tissue injury to the arm and thorax. The subject had been shot through a car window and fragments of glass and shot are shown in the soft tissues.

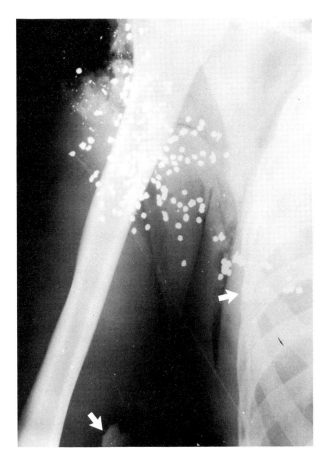

energy from missile to bone. Bone fragments then become themselves injurious objects. They may sometimes emerge from the body and cause doubts as to the nature of the secondary injury.

As an example, one author was called to a shooting incident involving a boy, where two cleanly-incised wounds on the back of the neck prompted detective officers to wonder whether the boy had been stabbed before being shot. The entrance wound of the shotgun was on the front of the neck and radiology as well as dissection, revealed numerous sharp fragments of shattered cervical spine lying in the tissues. The fragments were incomplete and it was obvious that the two cleanly-cut skin wounds were in fact exit wounds of sharp fragments of cervical vertebrae which had been blown outwards through the skin (Fig. 4.6). Fragments of glass may embed themselves in the soft tissues particularly if the missile has been discharged through a window (Fig. 4.7).

As well as its use in acute death, radiology of firearm wounds may have value long after the actual discharge has taken place. In a number of cases, bullets or fragments of shot have been detected radiologically many years after injury, which includes war wounds. Several cases involving claims for disability pension following war service and civil actions for damages following some accidental discharge, have been clarified by radiology of the affected part, which may reveal definite proof—or lack of proof—of such metallic projectiles in the tissues.

Occasionally, radiology can assist in confirming the nature of an obscure injury, which may or may not be a firearm wound. On a number of occasions, a distant firearm wound has been confused with a stab wound or penetrating lesion from some other weapon. Radiology has been the first means of confirming that there are metallic projections within the tissues and revealing the true nature of the injury. In a recent case, one author was presented with a skull of fairly recent origin, hidden in a rubbish dump. The skull had a circular defect in the right frontal area and because of slight scalloping of the edges, the possibility of a shotgun blast was considered. No naked-eye shot or metallic fragments could be seen, but radiology revealed tiny flecks of metal embedded in the margins of the bone defect and also embedded in the inner table of the skull on the opposite side to the entrance wound. The fragments were minute, being embedded in the bone and virtually invisible to the naked eye, but radiology was sufficient to confirm the true nature of this obscure injury.

Bombs and explosives

Much of what has been said concerning firearm injuries is applicable also to injuries from explosive devises. Regrettably, the incidence of injuries and deaths from bombs has greatly increased due to urban terrorism. In these cases, the size of the device is much smaller than those used in conventional warfare and hence most deaths and severe injuries are due to mechanical trauma from fragments either of the bomb or surrounding materials, rather than to blast injuries. In terrorist situations, blast injuries sufficient to cause death are rare except in the immediate neighbourhood of the bomb, usually so close that the common victims are those actually planting the bombs. This means that most injuries will be accompanied by fragmentation and embedding of fragments in the tissues.

In the clinical situation, radiology will naturally be of prime importance in the direction of surgical treatment. Here it might be pointed out that foreign objects seen on radiography might be of prime evidential value, especially to the investigating officers who are seeking the origin and manufacturers of the explosive device. Thus the X-rays and the foreign material if subsequently removed at surgery may be of great value to the law enforcement authorities. They should be retained and any unusual objects such as springs or pieces of metal or plastic which may be part of the detonating or timing device offered to the investigating officers.

Exactly the same considerations apply in autopsy work on bomb victims. Radiography is essential and even the most prosaic artifacts seen and recovered from bodies and their surroundings may be of considerable value in the investigation of the outrage. As an example, the originally unexplained crash of a Comet aircraft into the Mediterranean many years ago was due to an explosive device and particles in a body and in seat cushions were identified by radiography and assisted in confirming that a bomb had indeed caused the accident. In Ulster and on the mainland of the UK some cases have revealed metallic foreign bodies which have proved to be parts of the mechanism of the explosive device, and have assisted the authorities in identifying the likely manufacturer.

In deaths and injuries from bombs, the foreign bodies may arise directly from the casing of the device, from adjacent objects which have been scattered by the explosion or from falling masonry or other structures which have collapsed due to the explosion. Radiology followed by careful dissection may help to categorize these foreign bodies and assist in reconstructing the circumstances.

Where death has been due to the direct effects of blast, usually in more military situations, then radiology may show specific lesions, especially at interfaces in the body between tissues of different density.

Blast injuries

Injury to blood vessels may develop as a direct result of bomb blast as illustrated in Fig. 4.8 (a–b). This patient was admitted with a penetrating head wound and multiple facial lacerations. A pulsatile swelling in the left axilla developed later. Arteriography showed obstruction of the left axillary artery with a false aneurysm.

Bomb blasts, especially high-energy military devices, can produce extensive abnormalities in the lungs. The side nearest the blast is usually mainly affected as shown in Fig. 4.9. Extensive consolidation is shown extending outwards from both hilar regions, more marked on the left side. It should also be pointed out that major changes can and do develop on the side away from the blast. It usually takes about 6 hours

Fig. 4.8. (a and b). Presented with a penetrating head wound following a bomb explosion. Later developed a pulsatile swelling in the left axilla. Arteriography showed obstruction to the axillary artery and a false aneurysm was present.

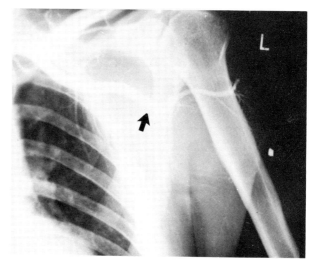

(a)

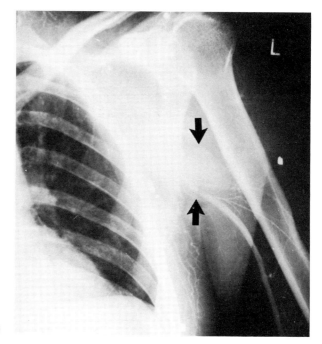

(b)

after the injury for any radiological abnormalities to develop. The radiological changes result from exudation of oedema fluid and blood into the lungs and interstitial tissues.

Fig. 4.9. There is diffuse consolidation in the left lung and patchy consolidation in the right lung following involvement in a bomb blast.

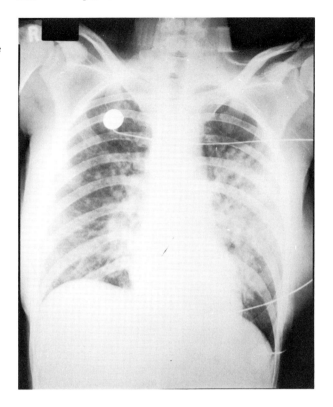

Foreign bodies

Apart from those arising from weapons and explosives, the impaction of foreign objects within the body is relatively commonplace, both in clinical practice and in autopsy work. In non medico-legal situations, foreign bodies may be inhaled, thrust into virtually every orifice of the body or even directly into the tissues. Children, mental defectives, sufferers from various perversions and victims of assaults may all have foreign objects, which are commonly radio-opaque, impacted within the body or its cavities. Radiology may be vital in the detection and localization of such objects, and play a prime role in directing their surgical removal.

Children may insert objects, including playthings, into nostrils, ears and especially the respiratory or alimentary tract. These objects vary from lead pencils to Dinkie toy cars, from glass marbles to coins. Where they have entered the oesophagus or stomach, radiological survey may be necessary to decide whether their size and shape may allow excretion through the normal channel or whether surgical intervention may be required. In children, objects frequently enter the trachea and again radiology may be vital for the evaluation of best means of extraction.

These cases rarely have medico-legal aspects, except where allegations of negligence may arise at a later date and the radiologist may find himself assisting in the proof of the occurrence. Medico-legal problems are more likely to arise in various forms of perversion. Foreign bodies are not infrequently introduced into the urethra, of both males and females and a wide variety of artefacts may become impacted in the urethra or bladder as a result of this peculiar habit. Pencils, even pencil cases, nails, pieces of catheter and other objects which are usually radio-opaque may be detected in this way by radiology. Again the major aspect is therapeutic rather than medico-legal, but some cases may eventually have forensic connotations. The author has seen several instances where objects were impacted into the rectum, some cases by the patient himself, but in two instances as a result of a homosexual dispute. Glass tumblers, large potatoes, pieces of broomstick, etc, have been inserted high into the rectum and even colon and here radiology may be a necessary adjunct to surgical removal. Where these cases end in a charge for assault, indecent or otherwise, then the radiological findings may form part of the evidence. In heterosexual assaults objects may be forced into the vagina and a recent case involved a fragment of broken glass, which had been used to scar the body of a murdered girl, before being introduced into the vagina. Fragmentation of such objects and penetration of the tissues may require radiological survey to determine their number and position.

Where the foreign object is in the soft tissues, rather than in a body orifice or cavity, then radiology may form an important part of both therapeutic and evidential investigation. In traffic accidents, foreign bodies are frequently impacted in the tissues, and may be found almost accidentally at autopy unless radiology has been performed where there are penetrating external injuries. The author has seen a complete door handle from a Renault motor car embedded deep in a liver, having been snapped off as the vehicle struck the victim a glancing blow. There was a small penetrating injury in the lateral surface of the trunk with some paint flakes on the clothing adjacent to the defect in the clothes. Radiology revealed a curved piece of metal about four inches long which was later retrieved at autopsy.

Similarly, the winged 'A' emblem forming the bonnet mascot of an early postwar Austin car was discovered in the depths of the brain, having penetrated a relatively small scalp and skull wound. Radiographs of this particular case were striking in the extreme, as the totally radio-opaque emblem produced a startling appearance on the film.

A case occurred in the psychiatric wards of a Welsh general hospital in which a schizophrenic repeatedly opportuned medical staff about a piece of metal in his brain. This might well have had medico-legal aspects if radiology had not been performed. As the patient appeared much as usual, and showed no external signs, no notice was taken for some time, but eventually, largely to humour the man, a radiograph was taken of his head, when a nail file was found to be lying horizontally across both frontal lobes! The patient had manually pushed the nail file through the side of the forehead and through the thin temporal bone with apparently no ill results, a small external wound healing up unnoticed. Surgical removal was performed, the patient appearing neither better nor any worse after the experience.

Where medical and surgical malpractice is alleged, it is obvious that radiology frequently plays a considerable part, especially where retained objects following surgical operation are alleged. This matter has developed to such an extent that it is now standard practice to incorporate a radio-opaque thread into surgical swabs so that they can be readily visualized in the event of an errant swab being suspected. Radio-opaque markers in surgical swabs vary depending on the manufacturer and it is clearly important for the radiologist to be aware of this. A radiograph of surgical

Fig. 4.10. Metal markers in surgical swabs.

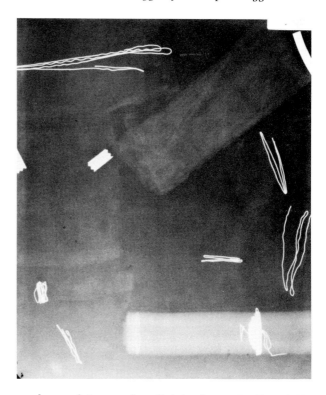

swabs used in one hospital is shown in Fig. 4.10. Surgical instruments (classically the Spencer-Wells forceps) are again obvious candidates for radiology in this context.

Where industrial accidents are concerned, radiology for foreign bodies frequently plays an important part. This may vary from the metallic or otherwise radio-opaque foreign body in the eye (which again not infrequently has medico-legal significance if it is missed clinically), to larger masses which may become impacted in the body as a result of an explosion. The latter may occur in many situations: a case is recorded by Usher where a pin holding two parts of a coalmining roof-support, was ejected by the pressure of the roof and flew like a bullet across the workings to penetrate the safety helmet of a miner and become embedded in his head with fatal results. Another case, illustrated in this chapter, concerned a mechanical explosion of a grindstone, fragments of which became embedded in the brain of the operator (Fig. 4.11a). Though once again most of the radiological aspects are concerned

Fig. 4.11 (a and b). Large fragment of grindstone embedded deeply in the brain following mechanical explosion. The relationship to the vascular structures is shown.

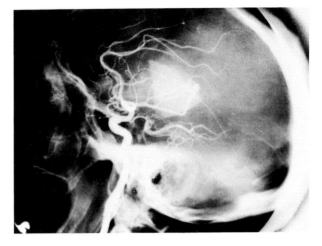

(a)

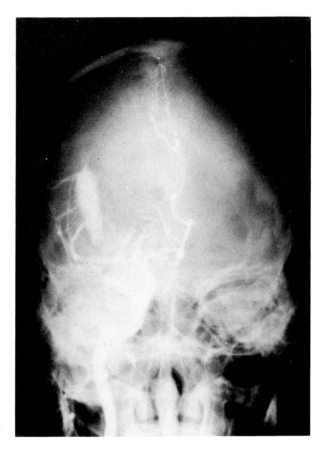

(b)

with the treatment and prognosis, they simultaneously become of considerable evidential value in matters of compensation and pension, sometimes even proceeding to civil litigation for damages for negligence against the employers. As with firearm injuries, the autopsy on such cases may be greatly facilitated by radiographic surveys carried out before the post-mortem examination, which will assist the detection, localization and enumeration of such foreign objects.

Head injuries

The radiology of head injuries is primarily for diagnostic purposes and the assistance and direction of clinical treatment, but the same films may later have medico-legal significance. This applies equally to post-mortem radiographs, and although direct exposure of the injuries is available at autopsy, radiography may be extremely useful where the damage is relatively inaccessible, especially in the facial bones where extensive autopsy dissection is only possible with the danger of disfigurement. The radiology of skull fractures may assist in the reconstruction of the type and direction of the impact, as an adjunct to autopsy demonstration.

In non-fatal cases or when death is delayed, radiographs of the initial lesions may provide similar information about the direction and severity of blows or impacts which have caused skull fractures, in cases where there is not necessarily surgical exposure of the affected areas, certainly not to the same extent as is possible at autopsy. Fissured fractures, 'pond' fractures and depressed areas of bone may be clearly revealed on radiology.

The complications surrounding the medico-legal necessity for radiology of head injuries is discussed elsewhere, but it might be mentioned here that although radiography is an extremely useful tool in head injuries, it not infrequently fails to demonstrate fractures, even of gross degree, particularly if it involves the base of the skull. In a recent case, a 14-year-old girl was struck by a motor vehicle and taken to a hospital casualty department. She died soon afterwards, but skull films taken before death revealed no fracture, only a fluid level in the sphenoid sinus, yet at autopsy there was a complete side-to-side fracture through the base of the skull passing through the pituitary fossa and effectively dividing the base of the skull into two separate halves.

The use of computerized tomography may have profound medico-legal significance in appropriate circumstances, as it is able to show focal lesions within the brain, irrespective of the visualization of bony damage.

Other internal traumatic lesions which may be revealed by radiography include air in the subarachnoid space where skull fractures communicate with the para-nasal sinuses or middle ear. Head injuries are fraught with forensic significance, especially in the sphere of medical negligence, where missed skull or brain damage later becomes the subject of litigation.

Fractures

The medico-legal aspects of trauma and orthopaedic surgery are legion and radiology plays a major role in the diagnosis and treatment and prognosis of such conditions. X-ray films figure largely in the evidence where such cases become the subject of civil or even criminal proceedings and are indispensable as evidence of the initial injury, the progress of treatment and the residual abnormalities, when taken in conjunction with the clinical assessment of the case. In autopsy work, radiology is not so important, as naturally direct exposure can be made in most cases. However, the whole body screening of suspected victims of child abuse is a vital preliminary to autopsy and is further discussed in the appropriate chapter in this book. Suffice it to say here that where an autopsy is to be carried out on a child with the slightest possibility of previous trauma, full body radiography should be performed before the autopsy, as the disruption caused by autopsy techniques tends to make interpretation of the films more difficult. Also, the pre-autopsy films are extremely useful in directing the attention of the pathologist to certain areas which might not normally be exposed, especially limb bones. The presence of injuries of different ages is vital and a whole spectrum of changes from acute fracture to fading callus may be seen. Similarly, where the indications are present, radiology of limb or facial bones may be extremely useful and blind dissection is to be avoided where possible. Evidence of old bone injury may be obtained more conveniently by radiography than by extensive post-mortem exposure.

A word of caution must be expressed at this point; there may be discrepancies in both directions when comparing radiography with the post-mortem demonstration of bones. In some cases, a radiographic suggestion of a fracture may not be demonstrable at autopsy dissection, no matter how thorough the latter may be. Conversely, fractures may occasionally be found by dissection which are not present on films of the relevant area. These discrepancies are fairly uncommon, but they do occur and the fact must be recognized in order to avoid prolonged and sometimes contentious medico-legal argument. It is more common for a fracture to be seen on dissection and not present on the films than the converse. Where a fracture has taken place with no displacement whatsoever, there may be physical factors which render the fine line of the break invisible on radiology.

Soft tissue injuries

The medico-legal implications of soft tissue radiography tend to be a spin-off from the clinical applications for diagnosis and treatment. In autopsy practice, it is less important, as the tissues may be examined directly, but in living patients, especially where later civil or criminal complications may arise, the demonstration of deep soft tissue injuries by radiography might be an integral part of the evidence. Mention has already been made of the visualization of intra-cranial and intra-cerebral traumatic lesions by CT scanning. By direct radiography, tomography or xerography, similar soft tissue lesions may be demonstrable in the subcutaneous tissues, muscle, and in the thoracic and abdominal cavity. Where these are traumatic, haematomata, abscesses, collections of fluid in serous cavities and air in similar cavities may all be demonstrable and may have medico-legal implications, especially where they are related to previous trauma.

Metallic poisons

Though an extremely rare occurrence, radiography may assist in detecting a suspected injection site where some metallic substance has been inserted into the tissue. Metallic mercury, antimony, bismuth and similar heavy metals are naturally densely radio-opaque and certain compounds of these metals, especially the oxides, may be sufficiently radio-opaque to be rendered visible by X-rays.

In less sinister, but also medico-legal circumstances, the escape of other radio-opaque substances into tissues where they ought not to be present, may be readily detected by radiography. Leakage of contrast medium from a blood vessel or escape of barium sulphate from the tract in which it was inserted for diagnostic purposes can be detected and evaluated radiographically. One such example was the escape of barium into the retroperitoneal tissues when an enema was being given to a patient with diverticulosis. A diverticulum ruptured and a large quantity of barium escaped into the tissues surrounding both the posterior, lateral and anterior aspects of the peritoneum. This particular case gave rise to medico-legal consequences for negligence.

Though really more appropriate in the section on foreign bodies, metallic objects at injection sites may be broken needles and again this is a situation not uncommonly associated with medico-legal consequences, where radiology can prove or disprove the allegations of a broken needle left in the tissues.

Closely related to the presence of metallic poisons beneath the skin, mention must be made of the metallic spheres criminally introduced into the tissues of two Bulgarian newreaders, one in London and one in Paris. The former died, because the metallic sphere, only 0·3

mm in diameter, was drilled to contain a minute
quantity of a toxic substance, probably from the castor
oil plant, Ricin. Though at autopsy the tiny projectile
was seen immediately adjacent to a small skin wound,
radiography may well have assisted if the foreign body
had penetrated deeply into the tissues instead of
travelling tangentially under the skin, as it did in the
non-fatal case in France.

Penetrating Wounds

Where deep penetrating wounds have been sustained,
the autopsy may sometimes be assisted by both direct
radiography of the wound, especially if air has entered
the wound and gained access to internal body cavities
such as pleura or peritoneum. Also contrast radiography may be performed by filling the wound with a
radio-opaque substance. This must be done only after
the wound has been fully examined for all its naked-eye
characteristics, then the introduction of a thick but
fluid contrast medium may be valuable in showing the
extent and direction of the track of the pentrating
injury. This is not recommended in cases where the
pleural or peritoneal cavity has been penetrated, as
naturally a large volume of contrast medium will
diffuse away from the original track and obscure any
significant appearances. The technique is most useful
in areas such as the neck, groin or surface of the limbs,
especially if the wound is relatively small, so that an
exact picture of the extent of the lesion can be obtained.
If the contrast medium solidifies after introduction, by
the incorporation of some gel, then the subsequent
dissection can frequently be assisted, as the solidified
cast of the wound can be employed as a core upon
which dissection can be centred.

  This technique should not be used if foreign bodies or
any trace evidence possibly present on the penetrating
instrument is likely to be in the depths of the wound, as
naturally the contrast medium will obscure and probably prevent the retrieval of such trace evidence. Direct
radiography should be carried out before the introduction of contrast medium, to determine whether any

radio-opaque fragments are present in the wound. The wound need not necessarily be due to a sharp instrument such as a knife, but may be due to all manner of objects. One author had such a case from a traffic accident in which a motorist collided with the back of a bus and a wooden stake, part of a bus seat, penetrated the wrist, emerged the other side and entered the thoracic cavity to perforate the left ventricle of the heart. Deep penetrating injuries can occur in any form of transport accident, whether road, rail or air and are frequently seen in industrial situations such as coal mines, steelworks and any other type of factory or building operation. In both fatal and clinical cases, radiology is an extremely useful accessory investigation, combined with all the normal surgical or pathological techniques.

Radiological manifestations of electrical injury

Electrical injuries result from the conversion of electrical energy into heat. The heat generated is proportional to the resistance of the tissues transversed. Individual tissues vary in their sensitivity to electrical injury and low voltage electrical current tends to travel along neuro-vascular bundles resulting in the death of such tissues due to avascular necrosis.

Vascular lesions were found in 6 of 11 patients after electrical injuries investigated by Hunt *et al.* (1974). Significant vascular abnormalities including complete arterial occlusions of an entire limb or a portion of a limb were found in 3 patients. They pointed out that partial vascular occlusion demonstrated by angiography did not accurately reflect the degree of tissue damage and amputation was often more proximal than could be predicted by the angiograms. However arteriograms can give valuable information in limbs with impalpable pulses. In such cases complete or partial vascular occlusion indicates muscle necrosis and the need for immediate surgery. A normal arteriogram was associated with only a 20% incidence of underlying muscle damage. It would appear that arteriography is of limited value as demonstration of small nutrient muscular branches is very difficult.

A case of thrombosis of the left renal artery secondary to an electric shock in a man aged 28 has been reported by Mogg (1977). Apparently he had been thrown to the ground having attempted to cut a live electric wire carrying 30 000 volts at the top of a pylon. He had been wrongly informed that the wires in the grid system were inert and that the grid was temporarily closed. Excretion urography showed a non-functioning kidney and aortography revealed complete occlusion of the left renal artery (Fig. 4.12).

Fractures of the 12th dorsal and 1st lumbar vertebrae following accidental electric shock in a 25-year-old man has been reported by Rajan *et al.* (1976). He developed severe pain in the back in the weeks following the incident and radiological examination disclosed fractures.

Pilling (1976) reports that it is standard practice in Sheffield to take radiographs of the footwear of the victims of fatal electrocution, to determine whether there are metal studs or inserts in the sole, which may have facilitated the earthing of the deceased through his feet to ground potential. Occasionally, the pattern of metal studs in working boots may be imprinted as actual electrical burns or localized zones of erythema on the soles of the feet, especially where damp or sweaty socks assist the passage of current. As some moulded rubber or plastic boots have metal reinforcing inserts hidden in their substance, radiography may help to match up these inserts with marks on the skin.

In radiological departments there are potential electrical hazards from failure to earth or inadequate earthing of radiological equipment. Sprawls (1971) has pointed out that when patients have pacemaker leads or catheters which can form a path for stray electrical currents directly to the heart, currents of approximately 100 μA can produce death. He described a study in which electrical currents flowing between the surfaces of X-ray machines, other equipment and grounded objects were measured in 29 X-ray rooms. Stray currents were found in 16 of these rooms to exceed hazardous levels for patients with cardiac catheters or exposed pacemaker leads. This arose

Fig. 4.12 (a and b). Thrombosis of the left renal artery following an electric shock.

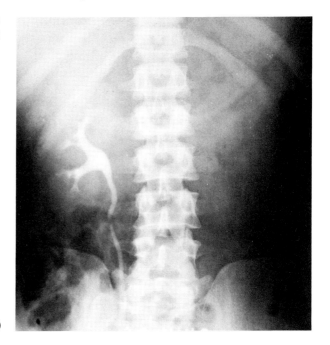

(a)

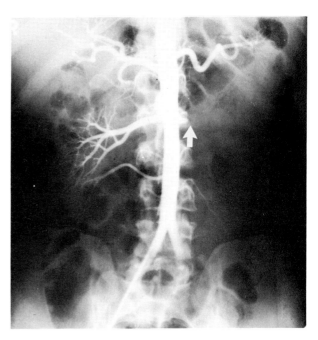

(b)

because the X-ray equipment was not securely grounded to a point which was at the same electrical potential as other grounded items in the area. To reduce the hazard Sprawls advised the installation of a marked common ground bus connected to earth ground through a rigid low-resistance path not in the circuit of the power distribution system. All pieces of equipment which have exposed conductive surfaces in the patient area should have their surfaces bonded to the common ground bus. The exposed portion of cardiac catheters and electrodes should be insulated against contact with other conductive objects.

Radiology in the diagnosis of drowning

Fatal immersion in water accounts for a very high toll of life annually, estimated as at least 140 000 each year on a world-wide basis, some 7000 in the United States and up to 1500 in Great Britain.

The number of 'near-drownings' is greatly in excess of the fatality rate, though no firm statistics are available. Hunter and Whitehouse (1974) point out that 'secondary drowning', i.e. deaths after the victim has been recovered alive from the water, is a problem of not inconsiderable magnitude, occurring at any time from minutes to several days after recovery from the water. In a series reported by Fuller (1963), 25% of 77 near-drownings died in the secondary phase. It is here that radiology may provide a useful method of assessment of the status of the patient and this occasionally may have forensic significance, both in subsequent civil and criminal litigation.

In experimental animals, the effects of inhaling salt water are markedly different from inhalation of fresh water. Inhalation of hypertonic sea water results in water passing from the blood into the alveoli. There is also a transference of electrolyte into the alveoli. Rapid haemoconcentration occurs and in human beings pulmonary oedema results. On the other hand inhalation of fresh water in experimental animals results in it being rapidly absorbed in to the circulation resulting in haemodilution and haemolysis of red blood cells.

However, Miles (1968) noted that the effect of inhalation of salt and fresh water are not so clearly distinguishable in human beings since complete investigations are seldom made during recovery. In cases where investigations have been made there has been no evidence of significant transfer of electrolyte and no haemoconcentration or haemodilution has been found (Fuller, 1963).

It is likely that water entering the lungs acts as an irritant and that this could lead to increased capillary permeability. In both fresh- and salt-water drowning, there is considerable loss of protein from the blood. Apart from the effect of inhalation of water, debris such as mud, sewage, and other pollution may also be inhaled. These may be responsible for subsequent clinical deterioration after an initial period of improvement.

Radiological manifestations

The radiological features vary. Putnam *et al.* (1975) found that the chest radiographs were initially completely normal in some patients, despite severe hypoxia. In other patients abnormal radiological signs did not develop for 24–48 hours. Characteristic findings are those of pulmonary oedema with diffuse opacities extending outwards from the hilar regions with relative sparing of the peripheral portions of the lungs (Fig. 4.13). There is no obvious difference in the radiological findings whether the victim was submerged in fresh or sea water (Rosenbaum *et al.*, 1964). The aetiology of the oedema is thought to result from prolonged hypoxia. In some fatal cases although the initial chest films were normal the patients later developed respiratory distress due to aspiration pneumonia. Usually the radiological abnormalities resolve within a few days but in aspiration pneumonia the lesions may be slow to clear.

Pulmonary interstitial fibrosis has been observed in an investigation which followed near drowning in fresh water. This was attributed to incomplete resolution of the alveolar interstitial pathology secondary to

Fig. 4.13. Diffuse pulmonary oedema in a case of drowning.

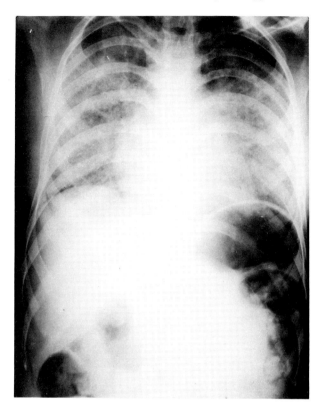

the near drowning and exposure to high oxygen mixtures.

Radiological evidence of sand aspiration in drowning and near drowning has been described by Bonilla Santiago *et al.* (1978). Early detection is important so that bronchoscopic removal can be attempted.

Vertebral artery trauma

During the past two decades, forensic pathologists have drawn attention to a hitherto undescribed cause for traumatic subarachnoid haemorrhage. Though the vast majority of subarachnoid haemorrhage is due to natural causes, either a rupture of a berry aneurysm of the Circle of Willis or rupture of an apparently normal cerebral artery, a number of cases were associated with trauma to the head or neck in which no berry aneurysm nor any bleeding point within the intra-cerebral course of the arteries could be discovered.

A number of workers (Contostavlos, 1971; Simonsen, 1976; Voigt, 1961; and Cameron & Mant, 1972) described injuries to the vertebral artery as it passes through the foramen in the transverse process of the atlas vertebra, giving rise to subarachnoid haemorrhage from tracking of blood from the damaged vessel through the foramen magnum. In most of these cases, there was a fracture of the transverse process of the first cervical vertebrae and the lesion has come to be known as the 'CV-1 syndrome'.

Radiology plays an important part in the detection of this rather occult lesion. The delay in recognizing the condition was due partly to the fact that this area of the neck is rarely examined at routine post-mortem and the superficial signs of injury may be slight or absent, being confined to bruises or abrasions on the neck or head, often at the level of the base of the skull.

Direct radiography of the area rarely reveals the fracture of the transverse process of the atlas vertebra and special techniques must be employed. These consist of (a) radiology of the excised upper spinal segment or even the isolated atlas vertebra and (b) post-mortem arteriography of the vertebral system.

The syndrome often has serious medico-legal consequences, as death may be the result of an assault leading to charges of manslaughter or even murder, and the requisite medical evidence must be obtained with the maximum detail and surety.

A detailed scheme for evaluating vertebral artery trauma has recently been published by Vanezis (1979). Radiography plays an important part in this suggested technique. At post-mortem, the neck structures are exposed by a standard post-mortem procedure and the tongue, larynx, oesophagus, etc, are reflected forwards. The origin of the vertebral arteries are exposed where they arise from the subclavian vessels. The calvarium is next removed and with the brain *in situ*, the basilar artery is ligated as close to the fusion of the vertebral arteries as possible. The calvarium is replaced, and injection of the vertebral arteries with contrast medium is carried out. It is recommended that a mixture described by Moller is used, consisting of barium sulphate sulphate suspension (0·6 g/ml), 15 g of gelatin and 2–3 g of gum arabic. The mixture is placed in a hot water bath until liquified, then injected into one vertebral artery with a syringe having a piece of PVC tubing attached. Approximately 5 ml of the contrast medium are sufficient. The mixture should be seen to emerge at the origin of the other vertebral artery, unless there has been severe trauma to one of the vessels, in which case it will leak into the tissues.

The neck is then either X-rayed *in situ* or the cervical spine is removed, preferably with the base of the skull surrounding the foramen magnum, being radiographed as a separate tissue block. Radiographs of excised neck specimens are usually of superior quality. An anterior–posterior view, a lateral and two oblique views are normally taken. Macro-radiographic views may also be employed to show smaller vessels in greater detail. The angiographic techniques reveal the point of damage to the vertebral artery and may show leakage of contrast medium into the tissues if there is a substantial rupture.

These injuries may be seen in the battered child syndrome, due to whiplash injuries caused by severe shaking. In adults, the commonest situation in which traumatic sub-arachnoid haemorrhage occurs follows a drunken altercation in which the victim is struck or kicked at the side of the neck, often at the level of the base of the skull.

In addition to these angiographic techniques, radiography may reveal a fracture of the transverse process of the atlas vertebrae, either a comminuted fracture passing into the foramen transversarium or a fissured fracture of the tip of the transverse process. Though this in itself does not damage the vertebral artery, it is a good indicator of trauma to that area of the neck, which in itself can cause damage to this major vessel, leading to massive subarachnoid haemorrhage.

Air embolism and pneumothorax

The autopsy diagnosis of air embolism is notoriously difficult and a number of cases are on record where, although clinical confirmation of air embolism was present, no air could be demonstrated at autopsy. Radiology is of great help in assisting the pathologist to come to the correct diagnosis and it should be routine for radiography of the head, neck and thorax to be carried out in any case where air embolism is suspected. Once the tissues are opened and veins breached, then it is extremely difficult to confirm air embolism by gross anatomical dissection.

Radiography with the correct penetration will reveal bubbles in the venous system including the great veins of the neck, the inferior *vena cava* and in the heart— both in the atria and ventricles when other more direct methods may fail to demonstrate such embolism. It is possible that air in the vascular system may decrease or may be completely absorbed in the post-mortem interval before autopsy is carried out, and radiography at or soon after the time of death may be a valuable and perhaps the only evidence of substantial air embolism.

It has recently been suggested that air embolism may be more frequent than is suspected after surgical intervention and that deaths during or soon after surgical operation should be routinely radiographically screened to exclude the presence of air embolism. A recent case in which fatal air embolism followed vacuum aspiration for termination of pregnancy showed unequivocal air embolism radiologically but nothing could be demonstrated by the most careful autopsy (Fig. 4.14). In all cases of suspected death from criminal abortion, such radiographic screening should be carried out and probably in the extremely rare case mentioned above, where uterine vacuum aspiration has led to fatal results. Deaths after open heart surgery and after surgical operations upon the neck, such as thyroidectomy, are also obvious candidates for radiological screening to exclude air embolism. Penetrating injuries, especially of the neck and thorax are other conditions in which air embolism may not be demonstrable by any other means.

The hazards of deep sea diving have unfortunately become more evident in recent years. The dangers are well illustrated in the following series of radiographs of a young man who had been diving from a bell at approximately 100 m depth in the Celtic sea. He had

Fig. 4.14. Chest radiograph showing air within the heart, right main pulmonary artery and intra-pulmonary branches following vacuum aspiration for termination of pregnancy.

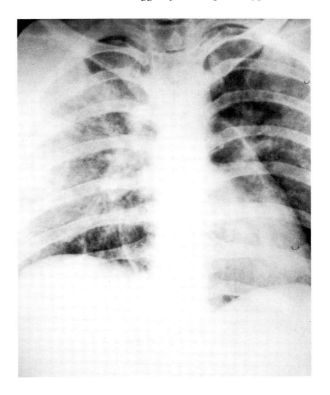

become distressed but during his attempt to re-enter the bell his life and air lines were inadvertently cut by a colleague. The bell with the dead man was brought rapidly to the surface and the deceased was consequently decompressed. At autopsy subcutaneous crepitus was palpable over the lower neck. Radiographs showed gas presumably nitrogen in the heart and major neck veins (Fig. 4.15).

Though the post-mortem demonstration of a pneumothorax is less difficult than that of air embolism, especially if it is a tension pneumothorax, radiology again offers a much better means of detecting both the presence and the extent of air in the pleural cavities. Where the clinical history suggests a pneumothorax, radiology is advised before autopsy dissection. Penetrating injuries of the chest are also candidates for such investigation as where there is no tension in the pleural cavity, it may be much more difficult to identify positively the presence of a pneumothorax on more autopsy inspection. Pneumoperitoneum is a similar

Fig. 4.15. Gas in the neck veins and heart in a deep-sea diver who had his life and air lines cut at 100 m depth.

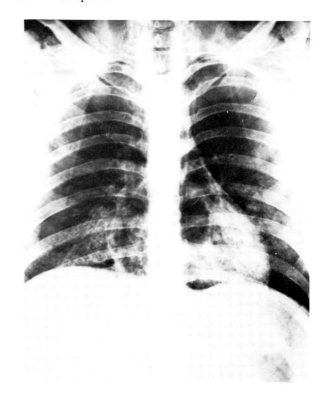

condition in which air or gas in the peritoneal cavity may be visualized radiologically more readily than by gross inspection, though the probable fatal complications tend to be less, the condition merely being an indicator of some defect in the continuity of either the gut or the abdominal wall.

Laryngeal injuries

Damage to the larynx has particular medico-legal aspects, as this is one of the areas in which homicidal strangulation frequently leaves evidence of trauma which may be of vital importance in criminal proceedings. The three main types of damage which occur in pressure on the neck are

(a) Fracture of the hyoid bone
(b) Fracture of the thyroid cornuae
(c) Fractures of the thyroid and cricoid cartilages.

The first one is the most well known but is rare except as a result of direct trauma such as manual strangulation, hanging or direct blows to the neck. The hyoid bone consists of a body and two paired processes, the greater and lesser cornuae. Fusion of the greater cornuae with the body of the hyoid is very variable and in the authors' series of 110 excised hyoids complete fusion with the body occurred in 39 subjects and partial fusion in 14. Fusion had occurred in one small subject aged 18 whereas at the other end of the scale no fusion had occurred in some subjects in the 8th and 9th decades. In many hyoids the greater cornuae were freely mobile and actual synovial joints were present. The young hyoid bone tends to be supple and bends rather than snaps under pressure and it is rare for fractures to be seen in adolescents. Clearly a hyoid bone with freely moveable joints with the greater cornuae would be much less likely to fracture than one firmly united. Examples of fused and unfused greater cornuae are shown in Fig. 4.16(a–b).

It is generally believed that removing the larynx at autopsy in itself may cause a fracture of the hyoid bone particularly in an older person. However, in the series of 91 excised hyoid bones referred to above none showed evidence of a fracture. It is usually held that to aver that a fractured hyoid was sustained during life, a haemorrhage must be demonstrated at the fracture

Fig. 4.16. (a) Unfused greater cornuae, hyoid. (b) Uni-lateral fusion greater cornu.

(a)   (b)

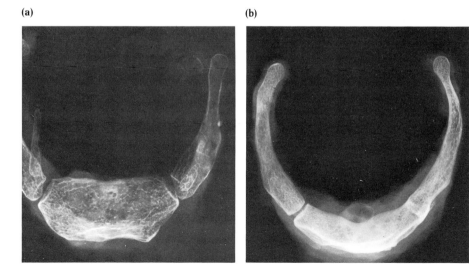

site. However on occasions this may not be true, as some fractures do not bleed at all, even when examined microscopically and post-mortem seepage from a fractured bone may cause a small haemorrhage even after death.

Radiological examination of the larynx *in situ* to detect the presence or absence of a fracture can avoid subsequent accusations that dissection may have caused an accidental post-mortem fracture. The larynx can be examined in the antero–posterior and lateral positions and if the larynx is excised *en bloc*, further radiological examination including tomography may provide additional valuable information regarding the presence or absence of a fracture in the laryngeal cartilages.

Of course, the radiological demonstration of a hyoid fracture does not indicate that it was caused during life, but the value of radiology is that examination of the laryngeal structures can be made before manual interference is carried out by the examining pathologist. In addition, the fine structure of the laryngeal structures and an exact demonstration of any damage can be readily obtained in a convenient form for examination at any later date up to and including exhibition at a criminal trial. Microradiology has been carried out by Kunnen *et al.* (1976) in homicide cases.

The cornuae of the thyroid cartilage are very similar to the greater cornu of the hyoid bone and may become fractured in almost exactly the same way. It has been said that fractures of both the greater cornu of the hyoid and of the thyroid cornuae are frequently caused not by direct pressure on the prominences themselves, but due to traction by the attachments of the thyrohyoid membrane which extends between the pairs of cornuae. Where a strangling hand is placed on the neck, the fingers may indent this membrane and the subsequent shortening and traction may cause torsion and stress to breaking point, especially or perhaps only if calcification is present. Fractures of the thyroid cartilage or plate itself are always due to a blow on the larynx, rather than pressure from strangulation.

A blow either to the side or front of the neck, as in the

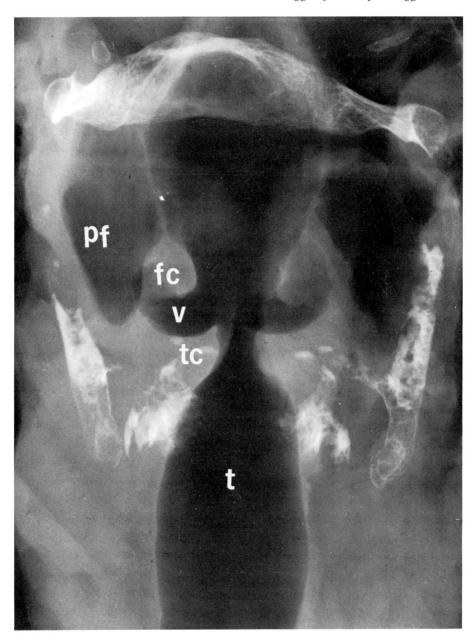

Fig. 4.17. Radiograph of an excised larynx from a case of hanging. Note the clear demonstration of the normal anatomy. pf (pyriform fossa), fc (false cord), v (ventricle), tc (true cord) t (trachea). No abnormality shown.

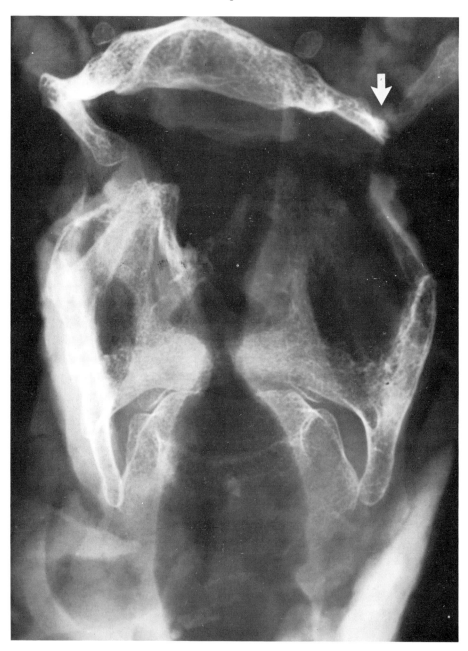

Fig. 4.18. Fracture of the hyoid
bone following hanging.

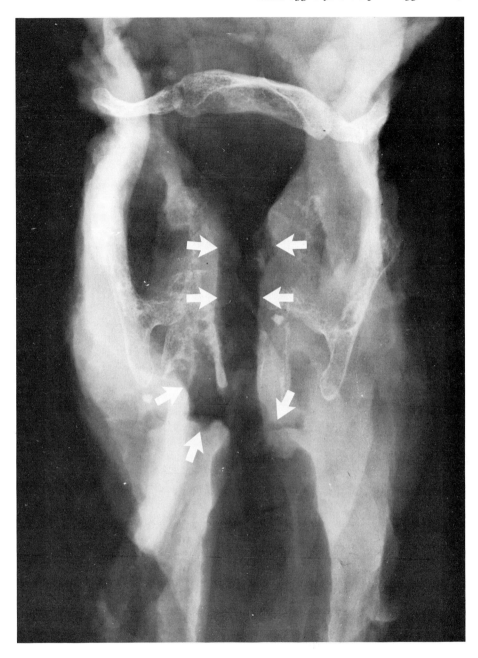

Fig. 4.19. Gross narrowing of
the supra-glottic airway and
distortion of the larynx
following strangulation.

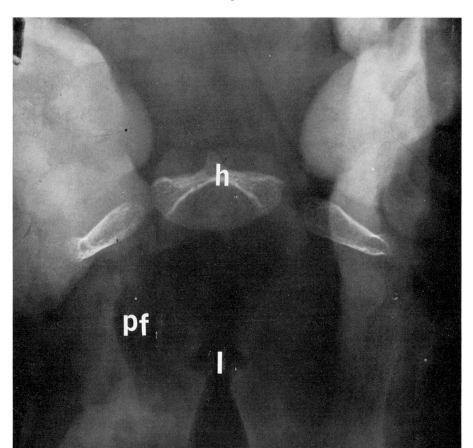

Fig. 4.20. Larynx of a child strangled by a ligature. No abnormality seen in this case. Presumably the mobile hyoid bone resisted fracture.

'Commando-punch' or 'karate-chop' may cause a linear fracture of the relatively large area of cartilage exposed. This was demonstrated in the Emmet Dunn murder in the BAOR in Germany, where a death originally certified after autopsy as being due to suicidal hanging, was shown on a later exhumation to be a commando-punch to the throat, causing fracture of the laryngeal plate.

Fracture of the cricoid ring, the upper ring of the trachea immediately below the thyroid cartilage, is relatively uncommon but may be seen in either a blow to the neck or very rarely to a strangling pressure which is applied much lower down the neck than is usual in manual strangulation. Rarely, a low ligature may also overlie the cricoid and cause a linear crack which is almost always in the mid-line.

Excellent detail of the larynx can be obtained with soft tissue radiographs taken in both the antero–posterior and lateral positions. Fig. 4.17 illustrates the normal anatomy of the excised larynx in a case of hanging. No fracture is shown in this case. On the other hand, Fig. 4.18 shows a fracture of the greater cornua of the hyoid bone in an elderly man found hanged. The soft tissues may show evidence of damage particularly in cases of strangulation. The supraglottic airway is markedly narrowed and the larynx itself is distorted in such a case (Fig. 4.19). No abnormality was found in the larynx of a child strangled by a ligature (Fig. 4.20). Presumably the hyoid bone was very mobile and bent rather than fractured as previously suggested.

5 Child abuse

It is only in relatively recent years that the entity of child abuse has been recognized though there has always been violence to children by parents and guardians. An increasing number of studies have now exposed the extent and gravity of the problem.

The vital role of radiological examination in the diagnosis of child abuse has become established since the description by Caffey (1946) of a syndrome in which fractures of the long bones were associated with subdural haematoma. Although there was no history of trauma in any of the cases described it was considered that the subdural haematomas were traumatic in origin and that the bone lesions were also likely to be the result of trauma.

Later the suggestion was made by Silverman (1953) that the syndrome described by Caffey resulted from mal-treatment by custodians. Further support for these ideas came from Woolley & Evans (1955) who stressed the hazardous conditions under which such children lived. The radiological appearance of the bones in the affected children were bizarre and unusual and presumably resulted from repetitive injuries either due to an unawareness or a deliberate denial on the part of those responsible.

Dramatically the condition was brought to the notice of the medical profession and the general public by Kempe (1963) who referred to the condition as the 'Battered Child Syndrome'.

The true prevalence of the condition is unknown but it is likely that the syndrome is still under-estimated. The report of the Committee on Child Health Services suggested a figure of not less than 5000 affected children a year in England. Seven to eight per cent of such children die and non-accidental injury represents the fourth commonest cause of death in the first five years. The report also stated that of those who survive 11% had residual brain damage and 50% visual impairment of varying degree.

Gil (1969) did not consider that 'battering' was a major social problem with an incidence of less than 7000 cases per year. On the other hand Kempe (1971) estimated that there were 30–50 000 cases annually in the USA. He indicated that roughly 25% of all fractures seen in the first two years of life were due to the battered baby syndrome.

Although child abuse is found in all social classes there appears to be an increased incidence in lower social brackets. Parents who abuse their children have frequently been subjected to abuse themselves. Gil (1969) has also identified certain psychiatric features. It appears that there is a rejection of the abused child and a reversal of the normal role so that the parent expects a response from the child which the child would normally receive from the parent. There is also an increased incidence in children with a low birth weight and there is some evidence to suggest that abused children are disagreeable personalities.

A history of trauma may not be forthcoming and as Cameron, Johnson and Camps (1966) have rightly observed, 'the skin and bones may tell a story that the child is either too young or too frightened to tell' and it is here that radiology can play a vital part in confirming the diagnosis of child abuse. Clinical examination may reveal evidence of neglect and the affected child is often unusually quiet and withdrawn. Various skin lesions such as bruises may be present or even human bite marks. Thermal or caustic damage may mimic other conditions and mucosal tears particularly in the mouth due to direct blows are sometimes present. Not infrequently no external marks of violence are evident. It has been estimated by Fontana (1971) that one out of every two battered children dies after being returned to the parents and that many of the survivors will show evidence of psychological and emotional disturbances in adolescence. There is often delay before children are taken for medical care unless they are acutely ill and the parents fear impending death. The history obtained from the parents is nearly always inconsistent with the findings on clinical and radiological examination.

The aetiology of some of the radiological and clinical findings in the condition has been considered in detail by Caffey (1972; 1974). He noted that many of the affected infants had no obvious external trauma or skull fracture despite the presence of intra-cranial bleeding. Caffey suggested that both metaphyseal avulsions and sub-dural haemorrhages might result by forcefully grasping the infants by the extremities or thorax and shaking them. The latter produces whip-lashing of the head on to the thorax and this movement is potentially more dangerous in infants than in older children, as the infantile head is relatively heavier and the neck muscles weaker. Such movements in small children with large fontanelles and open sutures results in excessive shearing forces occurring at the attachments of vessels to the more rigid soft tissues such as the *falx cerebri*. It was also considered that such trauma could well be an important cause of subdural haematomas and intra-ocular bleeding. This explanation could account for the presence of such lesions in the absence of signs of trauma to the head or fracture of the skull together with traction lesions of the periosteum in the absence of fractures. It was further proposed that whiplash shaking could also be responsible for repeated intra-cranial and intra-ocular bleeding which might be responsible for cerebral palsies, mental retardation or permanent impairment of vision.

RADIOLOGICAL FEATURES

Skeletal injuries

A carefully conducted radiological examination can disclose not only the aetiology of bone lesions but may give information regarding the approximate age, number and sites of bone abnormalities. Trauma in the growing skeleton provides an opportunity for the radiologist to play a vital role in the diagnosis as trauma is frequently unsuspected by physicians and surgeons and may not be considered unless a history of trauma is available. A search for more exotic causes to explain the symptoms is frequently undertaken. In this condition Caffey considers that the radiologist can safely disregard the clinical findings as these may be completely misleading. Traumatic lesions may be present in a number of bones and these may be of differing ages. If an unusual injury is found without an adequate explanation it is important to carry out a full skeletal survey.

In young children the periosteum is loosely attached to the underlying bone so that separation may occur with trauma. The periosteal blood vessels are torn and bleeding takes place under the periosteum stripping it off the cortex often for quite long distances. The periosteum is however, tightly attached to the end of the shaft and to the epiphyseal cartilage. These anatomical facts explain some of the radiological findings.

Injuries to the metaphysis

These may result from swinging the baby, forcefully wrenching or twisting the limbs. Fragmentation of the

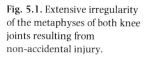

Fig. 5.1. Extensive irregularity of the metaphyses of both knee joints resulting from non-accidental injury.

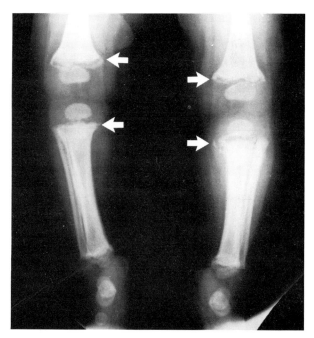

metaphyses may result from such trauma and these may be partially or completely separated from the end of the shaft (Fig. 5.1). These features can be seen on radiographs taken immediately after the injury and are pathognomonic of trauma whatever the cause (Caffey, 1974). Small portions of the adjacent cortex may also be detached and occasionally a portion or all of the provisional zone of calcification may be avulsed from the shaft. Generalized irregularity of the metaphysis may be shown.

Thickening of the cortex

The presence of a sub-periosteal haematoma results in separation of the periosteum from the underlying bone. The outer rim of this forms a thin bony shell 7–14 days after the injury. This bony shell rapidly thickens particularly near the ends of the shafts but often extends along the whole shaft (Fig. 5.2). Many of these

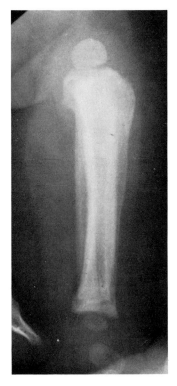

Fig. 5.2. Calcified sub-periosteal haematoma. Same case as shown in Fig. 5.1 some months later.

calcified sub-periosteal haematomata are lumpy with irregular margins. Occasionally the periosteal new bone extends around the metaphysis between the metaphysis and epiphysis producing the so called 'bucket handle' appearance (Fig. 5.3).

It is important to remember that long, smooth periosteal thickening is frequently present in the legs of newly born infants delivered by breech extraction and is sometimes shown in healthy full-term infants. This entity presumably results from normal handling and the periosteum elevates secondary to small sub-periosteal haematomas.

Late changes

When the proliferative cartilage in the contiguous epiphyseal cartilage is injured local maturation may be

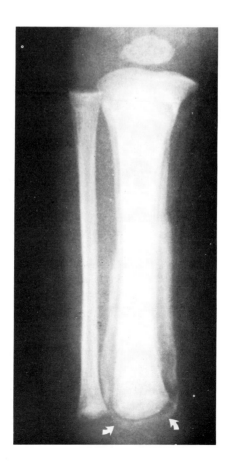

Fig. 5.3. Extensive periosteal thickening and elevation. The periosteal new bone extends between the metaphysis and epiphysis ('Bucket Handle' appearance).

accelerated and growth increase may occur presumably resulting from local hyperaemia resulting from the injury. The injury to the lower end of the shaft may result in a 'squared' appearance (Caffey,). It is likely to be due to fusion of metaphyseal fragments to the lower end of the shaft in an irregular arrangement beyond the uninjured end of the shaft (Fig. 5.4 a–b).

The axis of growth of a shaft may be affected from displacement of the metaphysis and its attached proliferating cartilage. Direct injury to the epiphyseal cartilage results in impairment of the blood supply and cupping of the metaphysis results as the peripheral margin of the cortex continues to grow while there is retardation of longitudinal growth. Caffey (1946) has pointed out that injuries to the hands may simulate rheumatoid arthritis both clinically and radiologically.

Injury may produce separation of epiphyses and accessory centres may also develop, whereas injury to the cartilage could result in shortening of the shaft. Displacement of epiphyses may result in an alteration in the growth axis and permanent deformity.

Healing rib fractures are sometimes encountered in the new-born arising from peri-natal injury. Apart from this, rib fractures are uncommon in childhood and the presence of these in the absence of a history of trauma should make the radiologist very suspicious of child abuse. In such cases the rib fractures are usually multiple and are most frequently encountered in the posterior or lateral aspects of the ribs. Separation of the costochondral junctions may also occur and are particularly well shown when the lesions are healing. The anterior ends of the ribs in these cases show expansion and sclerosis (Fig. 5.5).

The ribs, like other parts of the skeleton, may show fractures at various stages of healing. Such fractures are frequently bilateral due to side-to-side pressure from adult hands grasping the child around the thorax and squeezing during shaking. Callus formation is sometimes striking, presenting as a 'string of beads' appearance in a vertical line down a number of ribs (Fig. 5.6).

Although epiphyseal/metaphyseal fractures form the classical radiological findings in infants suffering

Fig. 5.4 (a and b). Extensive injuries to both elbow joints resulting in permanent deformity.

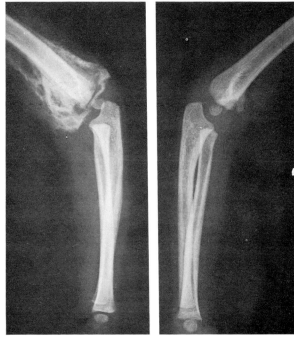

(a)

(b)

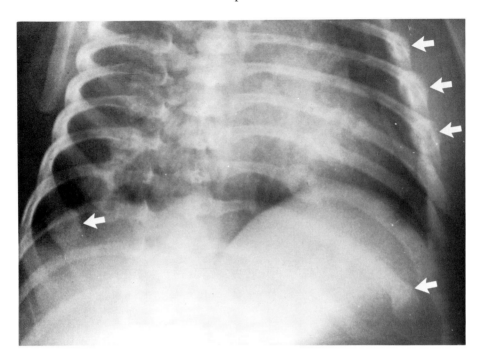

Fig. 5.5. Expansion and sclerosis of the costochondral junctions on both sides as well as posterior fractures.

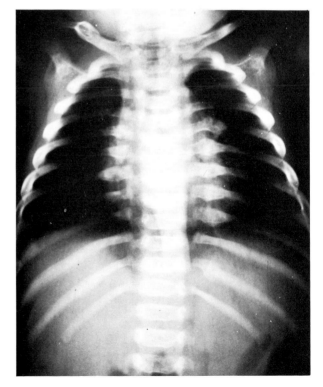

Fig. 5.6. Multiple fractures involving many of the posterior ribs on both sides with extensive surrounding callus.

from non-accidental injury, in one series of 100 children reported by Kogutt *et al.* (1974) spiral and transverse fractures of the long bones were more common. The mechanism of the injury was believed to be either from direct trauma or forceful twisting and wrenching of the limb. In the same series fractures in uncommon sites were encountered, including fractures of the lateral end of the clavicle. These are not usually encountered except as a result of peri-natal trauma or following child abuse. Such an injury is probably produced by shaking or twisting. Sternal and scapular fractures were also encountered and these should also arouse suspicion of non-accidental injury unless there is an adequate explanation to account for them.

Head and spinal injuries

A fracture in the parieto-occipital region is the commonest manifestation of a skull injury following a fall. In one series of 40 patients of child abuse 22% had skull fractures and in some of these there was associated sutural diastasis. Others showed sutural diastasis without a fracture. In most cases it is impossible to differentiate accidental from non-accidental injuries on radiological grounds.

In a series of 45 children with non-accidental injuries seen by James & Schut (1974) at the Children's Hospital of Philadelphia over a period of 13 months one died, a syndrome of motor hyperactivity developed in another, while mental retardation was subsequently seen in six others. It was pointed out that the presence of multiple fractures on skeletal survey was found in only two children. Sub-dural haematomas and cerebral oedema are the most serious and urgent complications of the syndrome and remains the main cause of death or permanent neurological damage. As emphasized by Caffey (1972) subdural haematomas may arise in the absence of obvious fracture or signs of external injury to the head. He emphasized the importance of whiplash injuries to the brain produced by shaking.

Sutural diastasis may arise as a result of cerebral oedema as illustrated in the following case of a $2\frac{1}{2}$-year-old male infant who was found at autopsy to have multiple abdominal injuries. A skull radiograph taken before death showed wide separation of the sutures but there was no evidence of a skull fracture or of a subdural haematoma. Skeletal survey revealed a healed fracture of the left 8th rib. (Fig. 5.7, a–b).

Spinal injuries with or without neurological damage are uncommon. Hyperflexion injuries are thought to be the most common. A variety of radiological appearances have been described including notching of the anterior aspect of a vertebra, compression of a vertebral body or a fracture dislocation. The latter would be unlikely to occur other than from severe purposeful injury.

Injuries to the spine may arise from forceful hyperextension. A child of 4 months was found dead in her cot. She had been admitted to hospital at the age of 5 weeks with a fractured skull, multiple rib fractures and a fractured humerus (Fig. 5.8, a–b–c). At autopsy the previous fractures had healed but there was a recent injury to the spine which consisted of a splitting of the disc between the 10th and 11th thoracic vertebrae. At the Crown Court the father stated that because the child was crying he had shaken her and then thrown her down on to her cot and then punched her in the back. This explanation according to the pathologist could not possibly account for the severe injury.

Abdominal injuries

In an investigation of childhood deaths following abdominal injury in the State of Rhode Island visceral injuries in battered children were found to comprise 25% of the total. The presence of abdominal signs and symptoms in a young child particularly if malnourished or showing evidence of bruising or unexplained bone injuries should alert the clinician regarding the possible traumatic cause of the symptoms.

Radiological examination in non-penetrating injuries of the abdomen can assist in demonstrating

Fig. 5.7. (a and b). Marked sutural diastasis due to cerebral oedema. A healing fracture of the left 8th rib is present.

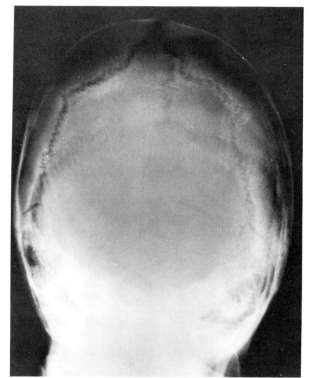

(a)

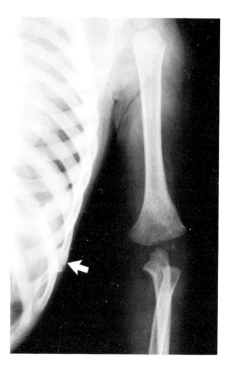

(b)

Fig. 5.8. (a) Extensive fissure fracture of the parietal bone. (b) Recent fracture left humerus. (c) Multiple rib fractures.

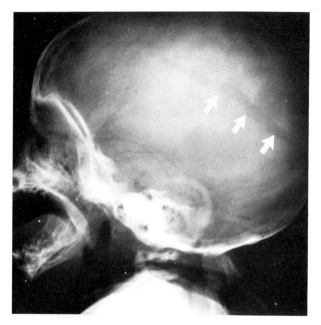

(a)

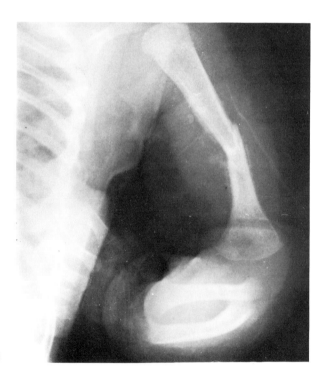

(b)

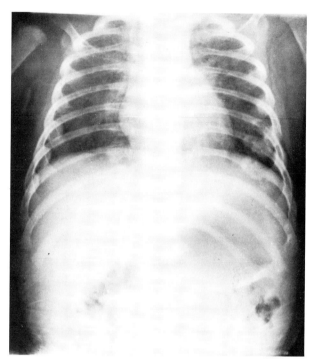

(c)

perforation of both intra- and extra-peritoneal organs. The liver, kidneys and spleen are most frequently involved. Injuries to the stomach, small intestine, pancreas and urinary bladder have also been reported. Plain films of the abdomen may reveal signs of free gas or fluid in the peritoneal cavity or signs of peritonitis. Retro-peritoneal haemorrhage frequently obliterates the renal and psoas margins or produces signs of a soft tissue mass. Meteorism, although a non-specific sign, can sometimes be helpful.

Rupture of the liver

Compression injuries to the thorax and upper abdomen may result in rupture of the liver and abnormalities of the thorax due to fractured ribs. Radiological examination may reveal associated pleural effusion, pneumothorax or surgical emphysema. The liver outline may be lost and there may be evidence of free fluid in the right flank.

The mortality from liver injuries is high and Camps (1969) reported 19 liver injuries in 100 fatal cases of battered children. Complete avulsion of the common bile duct from the duodenum has also been reported as a result of injury (Gornal *et al.* 1972).

Splenic rupture

The presence of splenic rupture should be suspected if fractures of the adjacent ribs are found. Enlargement of the splenic shadow together with a surrounding haematoma sometimes displaces the diaphragm upwards and the stomach medially. The presence of a splenic mass can be confirmed by introducing barium into the stomach and obtaining a radiograph with the patient lying on the left side. Radiographs of the abdomen showing an opacity with an even and straight lateral contour (Frimann-Dahl, 1960) is strongly suggestive of intra-peritoneal haemorrhage. The presence of sub-capsular haemorrhage is particularly important as this may rupture several days after the original injury. In cases where there is clinical and radiological doubt angiography is sometimes helpful in confirming the diagnosis.

Renal rupture

A history of haematuria in known or suspected injury suggests renal damage. Excretion urography is essential in such cases not only to assess the severity of the renal trauma but to establish the presence or absence of a contralateral kidney. This is particularly important in patients with severe injuries where surgery is contemplated. Arteriography is particularly helpful in assessing the viability of the kidney in severe injury.

Gastric rupture

Rupture of the stomach may result from blunt trauma. Radiologically signs of free gas are present in the abdominal cavity.

Injury to the small intestine

Serious intra-abdominal injuries due to blunt trauma following child abuse may be very difficult to diagnose in the absence of a history. Haller (1966) considered that injuries to the small intestine probably result from the retro-peritoneal fixation of the right part of the duodenum, and the fixation of the jejunum at the ligament of Treitz, so that these organs are compressed against the spine following blunt trauma to the upper abdomen. Complete transection of the duodenum or upper jejunum, haematoma in the bowel wall may also result due to blows to the front of the abdomen. Tears in the mesentery with associated retro-peritoneal haematoma, duodenal and pancreatic injuries were found in one autopsy series reported by Touloukian (1968) whereas McCort *et al.* (1964) found seven out of ten children with visceral injuries had rupture of the small intestine.

Intra-mural haematomas of the alimentary tract

It seems likely that most haematomas in the bowel wall arise from rupture of blood vessels in the mesenteric border of the intestine. However intramural haematomas have also been described in the muscular and sub-mucosal layers. Haematomas are most often seen in the 2nd, 3rd and 4th portions of the duodenum and proximal jejunum. Radiological examination may also show localized lesions due to bowel injury or obstruction producing proximal dilatation of the bowel. Occasionally the haematoma may rupture into the peritoneal cavity producing peritonitis.

Contrast examinations of the upper alimentary tract are very valuable in the diagnosis of intra-mural haematomas. Intra-mural masses, partially or completely obstructing the lumen, are characteristic while thick mucosal folds in the proximal loop of affected bowel and crowded folds distally produce a 'coiled spring' appearance simulating an intussusception (Fig. 5.9) (Stewart *et al.*, 1970).

Fig. 5.9. Characteristic mucosal changes in a patient with an intramural haematoma of the jejunum following trauma.

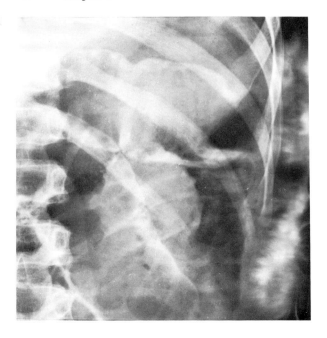

Injuries to the pancreas

Pancreatitis in children under the age of five is unusual and if present should always raise the suspicion of trauma. If there is no history of this a skeletal survey is advisable as this may show other manifestations of trauma.

Damage to the pancreas arises from compression against the upper lumbar spine by blunt trauma and if severe enough pancreatic enzymes are released into the lesser sac. These enzymes auto-digest the pancreas and surrounding tissues. As a result of inflammation in the lesser sac this becomes sealed by fibrous tissue and a pseudo cyst forms with clear yellow, haemorrhagic or purulent fluid within (Fig. 5.10).

Of thirteen children with proved pancreatic trauma seen at the Winnipeg Children's Hospital by Pena *et al.* (1973) nine were found to have a pancreatic pseudo-cyst. In three of these children under the age of three, child abuse was proved or strongly suspected. Pena and his colleagues suggested that where a pseudo-cyst of the pancreas was found and no acceptable explanation was available, child abuse should be considered.

Fig. 5.10. Traumatic pseudo-pancreatic cyst showing soft tissue mass in the upper abdomen with displacement of gas-filled bowel.

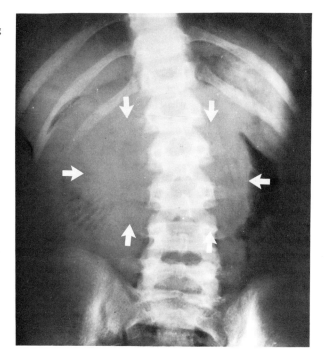

Pseudo-pancreatic cysts have also been reported in association with 'haemorrhagic' ascites, healing rib fractures or an associated haemorrhagic pleural effusion (Hartley, 1967). Although the association of a pleural effusion with pancreatitis is well recognized, a blood-stained effusion suggests traumatic aetiology. Kalwinsky *et al.* (1974) described the case of a three-year-old girl with ascites thought to be secondary to unsuspected blunt trauma.

The diagnosis of a pseudo pancreatic cyst secondary to trauma may however be difficult in young infants. The diagnosis should be considered in any young child with a palpable abdominal mass, abdominal pain, fever or abdominal distension (Bongiovi *et al.* 1969). Serum amylase levels are particularly valuable.

Certain radiological findings in localized trauma to the pancreas in children have been described by Young (1967). Straight radiographs may show increased density in the upper abdomen with localized paralytic ileus. The space between the gas-filled stomach and adjacent bowel may be increased. Examination with barium may show a coarse duodenal mucosa, sometimes with dilatation of the duodenal loop. Swelling of the head of the pancreas may produce enlargement of the duodenal loop (Fig. 5.11). The stomach and intestine may be displaced forwards. Ultrasonographic examination is probably the method of choice as not only may enlargement of the pancreas be detected but characteristic transonic masses are seen in cases with pseudo-pancreatic cysts.

Foci of fat necrosis in a number of organs have been found at autopsy in patients who have died of pancreatitis. Osseous lesions in pancreatitis have been described by Scarpelli (1956) in 10·4% of 67 patients with acute and sub-acute pancreatitis. The lesions within the bones may not appear for 3–6 weeks after the height of the clinical pancreatitis. Multiple punched-out osteolytic lesions in the long bones and the bones of the hands and feet are associated with cortical bone destruction and periosteal new bone formation. Later intra-medullary calcification may develop. The skeletal changes are painful and Slovic (1975) stressed that the findings may be similar radiologically to those found in leukaemia, sickle-cell infarction or metastatic malignancy.

Chylous ascites in a 20-month-old boy has been described by Boysen (1975). This is a rare manifes-

Fig. 5.11. Barium studies showing enlargement and distortion of the pancreatic loop in traumatic pancreatitis.

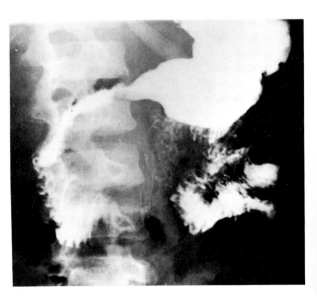

tation of child battering. A leak in the abdominal lymphatic system was demonstrated by lymphangiography and a skeletal survey showed healing rib fractures and a fracture of the right ulna.

The radiologist has an extremely important part to play in the diagnosis of non-accidental injury in children. It is important that the possibility of trauma, accidental or otherwise, should be considered in the differential diagnosis of vague or unusual illnesses in childhood. The finding of an unexpected fracture should be followed by a full skeletal survey. Infants referred with the clinical diagnosis of non-accidental injury should have each radiograph validated by the radiographer so that there can be no possible doubt in any subsequent legal case that the radiographs were those of the child in question.

Full skeletal surveys are important before autopsies on infants found 'dead in their cots' or found dying in mysterious circumstances. The pathologist will be alerted as to the possibility of child abuse if fractures are shown particularly if they are of differing ages.

There are a number of conditions that may mimic the radiological appearances of battered children and the following conditions may cause confusion:

Scurvy. Many battered children have been erroneously diagnosed as suffering from scurvy as minor injury in this condition produced large sub-periosteal haematomas. These rapidly calcified and eventually became incorporated with the underlying bone.

Radiologically and clinically the two conditions should be differentiated except in the rare cases where they coexist. In scurvy the bones show generalized loss of bone density whereas they are usually of normal density in battered children. A deficiency of Vitamin C gives rise to a true osteoporosis. A well-defined white line is present at the growing ends of the long bones (Frankel's line). It is also seen around the epiphyses and the carpal and tarsal bones. The zone at the ends of the long bones is abnormally brittle and leads to the production of micro-fractures. According to Gordon and Ross (1977) these are responsible for the formation of characteristic metaphyseal spurs (Fig. 5.12).

Fig. 5.12. Characteristic bone changes in scurvy. Note the osteoporosis, marked 'white line' at the metaphyses and a calcified sub-periosteal haematoma.

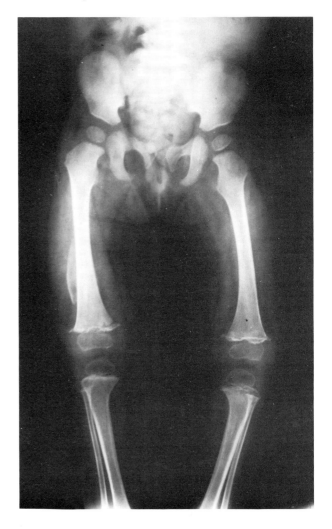

Osteogenesis Imperfecta. In this bone dysplasia multiple recurrent bone fractures arise after mild 'trauma but there is a marked variation in severity. Apart from the presence of fractures there is excessive tubulation of the bones which are usually thin and often markedly bowed (Fig. 5.13). The spine shows biconvex discs and basilar invagination is seen in the skull due to the bone softening. Multiple Wormian bones are characteristic. Bone formation is not deficient and abundant callus may be present around the fractures.

Congenital syphilis. Congenital syphilis may simulate the bone lesions of battered children and errors in

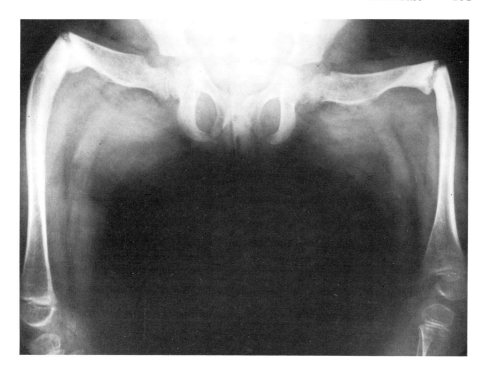

Fig. 5.13. Symmetrical
fractures with thin tubular
bones in a patient with
osteogenesis imperfecta.

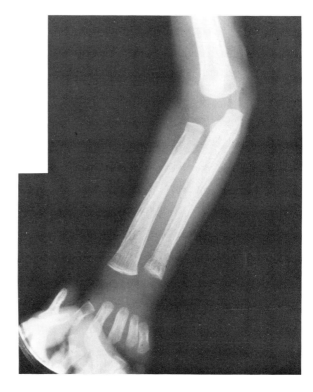

Fig. 5.14. Extensive periosteal
reaction involving the shafts of
all the long bones in congenital
syphilis.

diagnosis may arise (Fiser *et al.*, 1972). In both
conditions the periosteum may be elevated and thick-
ened (Fig. 5.14). However, in congenital syphilis the
lesions are usually bilateral and symmetrical whereas
trauma is often associated with asymmetrical lesions.
Congenital syphilis is now rare as routine serological
tests for syphilis are usually carried out in pregnancy.
The mother may, however, contract syphilis in late
pregnancy.

Infantile cortical hyperostosis. In this condition the
diaphyses of the bones are affected by extensive
periosteal new bone without bone destruction. The
mandible, ulnae, clavicles and ribs are most frequently
affected and in most cases the radiological signs
disappear by the age of three. The radiological and
clinical features are distinctive and should readily be
differentiated from the bone changes in the battered
child syndrome.

The Kinky Hair Syndrome. The radiological manifestations of the Kinky Hair Syndrome have been described by Wesenberg *et al.* (1969). They noted a
similarity to the battered child syndrome as periosteal
thickening of the shafts of the long bones were observed
and symmetrical metaphyseal spurring. Diffuse flaring
of the anterior ribs and Wormian bones in the skull
were also noted. They described malformation of the
intra-cranial arterial system and subdural effusions.
The similarity to the Battered Child Syndrome has also
been reported by Adams *et al.* (1974). There is evidence
that the major features of the disease are related to
copper deficiency.

6 Medico-legal implications of radiological procedures

OWNERSHIP OF RADIOGRAPHS

Radiographs are the property of the hospital or physician who took or caused to have them taken, to assist him in arriving at a diagnosis or in managing his patient. They do not belong to the patient, who has no legal right to their possession or indeed to a view of them.

However, the patient concerned certainly has an interest in them in a legal sense to the extent that they might be necessary for his future medical care or the protection of his legal rights. Any transfer of radiographs should be done via another doctor or medical institution and not through the patient or his legal representative. The films are part of the medical record of the patient and should be treated in the same way, having the same legal status as case notes. Where a film is required by another doctor or hospital for further treatment or management of the patient, the ideal course is to supply either a copy of the radiologist's report or a copy of the film, retaining the originals in the first location.

The matter is discussed by Bergen (1974) who recommends that the film or report should not be given to the patient, who is likely to misunderstand it or misinterpret it. The physician may feel obliged to give an account of the radiological result in terms understandable to the patient, but the legal ownership and physical possession of the film and report remain with the doctor. He should always be willing to supply another bona-fide medical attendant of the patient with all relevant information pertinent to further medical care or litigation. In the case of the latter circumstance, caution should be employed and the film or report transferred wherever possible to a medical expert nominated by the patient or his lawyer, rather than to the lawyer personally. All medical records, whether documentary or in the form of radiological or laboratory findings, should wherever possible, be confined to circulation within the medical profession rather than amongst lay persons.

OVER-USE OF RADIOLOGY

The demand for diagnostic radiological services has steadily increased and is currently growing at 5% to 10% yearly. Many radiologists are concerned about the increasing, expensive and often inefficient use that is being made of diagnostic radiological facilities. While the costs of radiological services increase, questions are being asked regarding the benefit to the patient from this work. Radiological examinations are the principal man-made source of radiation exposure.

There are a number of factors behind the explosion in the demand for radiological examinations. It appears that many physicians are moving towards defensive medicine partly due to the threat of litigation. Radiologists are also partly to blame by encouraging clinicians to refer their patients for radiological examination.

In Britain, it is now the view of the Department of Health and Social Security that the low incidence of pulmonary tuberculosis found in survey work no longer justifies the general need for mass radiography and the number of mass miniature units has been reduced. Furthermore there is little evidence that the use of screening techniques to detect carcinoma of the bronchus in asymptomatic patients affects the prognosis significantly. In any case the pick-up rate is only 0·27/1000 patients radiographed.

The chest radiographs of 1000 healthy children in New York were examined by Brill *et al.* (1973). They found that 6% of these were abnormal but the abnormalities consisted of minor skeletal lesions and none required treatment. They concluded that chest radiography should be considered on an individual rather than as a routine basis in children.

The value of pre-operative chest radiology has also recently been questioned. A multi-centre trial organized by the Royal College of Radiologists (1979) showed that of 10 141 study subjects 29·6% had a pre-operative film. The audit was restricted to non-acute non-cardio-pulmonary surgery. There was a three-fold variation in utilization between hospitals and marked variation in the utilization between various specialties. There was no obvious clinical reason for this. The study did not provide any evidence that a pre-operative chest radiograph influenced the choice of anaesthetic or the number who underwent general anaesthesia. There was also no evidence that the post-operative course was significantly different in those subjects radiographed.

It was concluded that pre-operative chest radiology should be used selectively where the clinical history or signs place the patient at high risk of post-operative pulmonary complication and where it is considered the investigation will provide important additional information. Routine examinations would also be justified in population groups where the incidence of undiagnosed chest disease is likely to be high, e.g. in immigrants.

Excretion urography is a time consuming and costly examination. Atkinson and Kellett (1974) commented on the large number of urograms in their patients with hypertension that were completely normal. They questioned whether treatable renal lesions were detected often enough to justify the investigations in all patients. They concluded that the highest yield of diagnosis for the lower 'cost' of renal investigations would be achieved if excretion urography were carried out on all hypertensive patients aged 40 or younger but only on older patients if there were a previously recognized renal abnormality.

Head injury is a common problem in infants and children. Mostly these are trivial but it is common experience that, irrespective of the severity of the injury, skull radiographs are considered mandatory in such cases if they attend hospital. There is considerable difference of opinion regarding the value of skull radiographs in the management of patients with skull trauma. It is clear, however, that the extent of the injury to the intra-cranial contents is of prime importance and the presence or absence of a fracture seldom affects treatment.

Roberts and Shopfner (1972) in a careful study analysed the clinical course in 570 children referred to their Department of Radiology for skull examination following trauma. A skull fracture was demonstrated in 49 (8·6%). There was no significant correlation between the incidence of fracture and symptoms neither was there any correlation between the type of fracture, the symptoms and physical findings. Furthermore, fractures located across the meningeal groove and sagittal sinus did not have a higher association with concussion, severe symptoms, sub-dural or extra-dural haematoma. An extensive study was also carried out by Bell and Loop (1971) to estimate the value and yield of skull radiographs in adult patients with skull trauma. They found no significant association of skull fracture with the clinical findings. It could be argued that skull radiography cannot be justified in the routine care of patients with skull trauma and that radiography should only be used if there is a possibility of a depressed fracture or foreign body.

Although abdominal radiography in pregnancy may be hazardous to the developing fetus, Carmichael and Berry (1976) found on analysis of the requests for abdominal radiography in a number of hospitals an overall incidence of 20% and in one of these over 35% of patients had radiography of the abdomen during pregnancy.

Diagnostic radiology properly applied is invaluable in the diagnosis of innumerable medical problems for which effective therapy exists. It includes reassurance that no abnormality exists. Pilling (1976) considered that indiscriminate use of X-rays could lead to real negligence as opposed to the spurious negligence which it seeks to eliminate. Doctors who order an X-ray in every case in which they think it could be asked for in court may be tempted to substitute the radiograph for an adequate clinical examination. Pilling concluded that if the young doctor is to give of his best, he needs an assurance that his conduct will be judged on its medical merits rather than by the traditional yardsticks adopted by the legal profession. Some studies of effectiveness point the way to a rational basis for control for what many call 'medical malpractice'. The threat of litigation could of course apply to patients who have been irradiated unnecessarily as well as those where radiology has been omitted.

The Medical Protection Society offered the following advice to its members in its 1975 Annual Report.

'Clinicians frequently assert that they order X-rays for medico-legal reasons when what they mean is that a fracture is not suspected but an X-ray is ordered simply to protect from possible litigation. To consider the relevance or otherwise of a particular investigation is to misunderstand the role of the Society and the value of membership to a particular clinician. Special investigations should be ordered only in accordance with an objective assessment as to what is clinically good and accepted practice in a particular situation.

'If, in spite of the careful exercise of clinical judgement, a mistake is made then the Society is glad to deal with the sequelae, whatever they may be.

'An appreciation of this attitude is unlikely to reduce the number of X-rays ordered, yet it is hoped that members will understand that they should feel under no pressure to practise defensive medicine to the ultimate detriment of patients or to feel that for their own safety, patients should be exposed to the potentially harmful effects that a full "*malpractice* check-up" could entail, such as is reported from the United States.'

In relation to the presumption of negligence when no radiograph has been taken following an injury, the Master of the Rolls, Lord Denning, said 'In some of the earlier cases the doctor had been criticized for not having taken X-rays with the result that they had sometimes been taken unnecessarily. This case showed that the Courts did not always find that there had been negligence because a patient had not had an X-ray; it depends upon the circumstances of each case.'

The case in question was Braisher versus Harefield

and Northwood Hospital Management Committee (C.A. July 13 1966). The case was quoted by Jellie; a similar opinion was expressed in a pre-war case, Sabapthi versus Huntley (1938, WWR 817).

The effect of diagnostic radiology on pre-natal development

There is widespread acceptance of the view that irradiation of the developing human embryo is harmful. Included in the recommendations of the International Commission on Radiological Protection (1977) is the following: 'because of the risk of radiation injury to any embryo or fetus the possibility of pregnancy is one of the factors to be considered in deciding whether to make a radiological examination involving the lower abdomen in a woman of reproductive capacity. Although such an examination is less likely to pose any hazard to a developing embryo if carried out during the "ten day" interval following the onset of menstruation attention should always be paid to details of radiological technique that would ensure minimization of exposure to any embryo or fetus that may be present whether or not the woman is known to be pregnant.'

The principle of the 'ten-day rule' has been accepted by the medical profession in the UK so that radiography of the abdomen in women of child-bearing age is not undertaken unless the patients are able to give an assurance that they are not pregnant. However, the doctor requesting an abdominal radiograph can decide to proceed if there are compelling clinical reasons not to postpone such an examination.

Conversely, a number of authorities in the USA (American College of Radiology, the National Council on Radiation Protection and Measurements in Report No. 54 (1977), the US Department of Health Education and Welfare (Food and Drugs Administration 1976), Brown (1976), Brown *et al.* (1976)) consider that restriction of irradiation to the first 10–14 days of the menstrual cycle is irrational since Graham *et al.* (1966) suggested that the ripening follicle may be as adversely affected by radiation exposure as the fertilized ovum. It has been argued that the least dangerous time for performing a radiological examination in early pregnancy might be between the 14 and 28 days from the first day of the last period.

In a very careful analysis of the risks Carmichael and Warwick (1978) concluded that there is no 'safe' period during which radiography of the lower abdomen of a women of reproductive capacity can be carried out but the evidence that irradiation pre-conception is likely to produce the same risks as post-conception is not confirmed.

Carmichael and Warwick stress that if a patient is pregnant UK practice would be to postpone radiography of the abdomen. They strongly recommend the continued application of the ten-day principle believing it to be an essential part of good radiological and radiographic practice.

The whole question of the ten-day rule should, according to Mole (1979), be reconsidered. He pointed out that the quantitative estimates of the various risks to the irradiated embryo or fetus have varying degrees of reliability. He estimated that the overall risk of serious radiation-induced harm following exposure of the developing embryo or fetus to diagnostic radiological examination in the first trimester of pregnancy is most probably in the range 0–1 cases/1000 receiving one rad tissue dose. The 0–1 cases would mostly be cancer in childhood. Severe mental retardation would be less common than cancer. The natural expectation for the birth of a markedly handicapped child at the end of a normal pregnancy is about 1/30. Mole suggests that concern over radiographic exposure of the developing embryo or fetus may be unnecessarily heightened by the existence of measures intended to reduce the possibility of exposure.

The argument is therefore unresolved but in the light of our present knowledge attempts should be made to reduce the radiation exposure to pregnant women in the reproductive period of life to the minimum.

Informed consent to radiological procedures

The legal concept of informed consent is exactly the

same for radiological procedures as it is for any other medical or surgical technique. However, there has been considerable recent controversy over the legal versus the medical indications for obtaining fully informed consent, this debate being particularly active in the USA.

To deal with the legal aspects first, the basic position is more firmly adhered to in Britain than in North America, where the American College of Radiology has issued a memorandum on the subject.

Basically, before any medical procedure is carried out, the permission of the patient must be obtained, this permission being valid only if the nature of the procedure has first been explained in comprehensible terms to the patient and he subsequently accepts it. To perform any physical procedure upon a patient without fully informed consent is technically an assault—or to be more accurate in legal terms, a battery. The patient may sue for damages in such circumstances, even if no physical harm ensued.

This concept of informed consent applies right across the board in medical practice. For uncomplicated medical procedures, such as the usual clinical examination involving palpation, percussion, auscultation, etc., the consent is usually inferred by the acquiescence of the patient, who has presented himself for diagnosis and treatment. This is often termed 'implied consent' and no special formalities are necessary. In ordinary clinical practice, this implied consent is often reinforced by the niceties of speech and common courtesy, such as a request by the doctor 'I would like to examine your chest, would you please open your shirt'. The tacit acceptance of this request is sufficient to form fully valid consent, though it may be difficult to prove at a later date if the patient becomes litigation-minded.

Again following the medical and surgical spectrum, more complicated procedures require 'express consent'. These range from vaginal or rectal examination to venepuncture or any of the more sophisticated and complicated diagnostic or therapeutic procedures. At a relatively arbitrary point along this spectrum of procedures, the consent, which is *express*, is usually obtained in writing and witnessed by an observer, so that any future dispute can be resolved by the production of a signed document. The presence of a document does not make the consent more or less valid in law, but is a convenient way of proving that such consent was obtained.

However, in recent years the concept of 'informed consent' has come very much to the fore, in which the necessity for explanation is an absolute prerequisite to the obtaining of valid consent. If consent is obtained by subterfuge or the glossing over of possible dangers, then the consent, whether documentary or oral, is invalid.

Recent changes in patient's attitudes and the general climate of civil and personal rights, has made it clear that every patient has a 'right to know' about his medical progress, including diagnostic and therapeutic techniques. He also has the right to know about the risks of any given procedure, so that he may decide whether or not he wishes to submit to such a procedure.

Though this is a convenient concept in legal terms, it is fraught with difficulties from the point of view of the medical practitioner. Almost every medical procedure has some element of risk and it then becomes a delicate matter to explain to the patient the necessity for carrying out the technique for the sake of his own health and the degree of risk which is inherent in the technique. In many instances, the degree of risk is very uncertain and cannot always be given with honest statistical accuracy.

Returning to radiological matters, all radiological procedures must be with the consent of the patient, assuming that he is mentally capable, adult and conscious. With straightforward procedures, such as chest or limb radiography, then the need for any substantial informing for the obtaining of consent is almost immaterial, as the risks of such examinations are virtually non-existent. Special cases such as radiography in pregnancy will be considered seriously by the radiologist and may require some explanation and decision on the part of the patient. When it comes to more complicated procedures such as the parenteral injection of contrast media, air-encephalography or

one of the many other complex radiological procedures, then this ranks equally with a surgical operation
and requires fully informed, written, witnessed consent. However, this concept which is one of legal
perfection, has been modified considerably by the
attitudes of American radiologists.

The great dilemma is in informing the patient of the
possible risks. Under the concept of 'right to know' then
the radiologist or other medical attendant should
discuss the matter with the patient and enumerate the
possible hazards of the radiological procedure. These
range from vascular damage when contrast medium
injected into an arm vein for a cholangiogram leaks
outside the blood vessel, to the possibility of paraplegia
from a myelogram.

When such complications are mentioned to the
patient, he may well take fright and although the risk is
relatively small, decide not to undergo the suggested
radiological procedure despite the fact that it may be
very beneficial to the diagnosis and treatment of the
ailment from which he is suffering.

It has been recommended that in discussing the
risks, an actual detailed list of the risks should not be
mentioned, but it should be stated that 'slight complications' or 'serious complications' might ensue. The
reasons for this is that though a doctor may list several
specific complications that might occur, he might omit
the very one that actually occurs in a given patient, in
which case the patient may sue on the grounds that he
was not informed of this particular risk.

Opinion amongst radiologists, especially in the USA,
is divided over the concept of informed consent. Hinck
and Wagner (1970) have summarized the matter,
indicating that it is the individual who performs a
diagnostic radiological procedure who is ultimately
responsible for obtaining informed consent. In obtaining consent, the patient (or his next-of-kin if he is a
minor or otherwise not legally responsible) should be
told what the procedure involves and what hazards are
entailed. The magnitude of the risk should be defined in
broad terms and the potential benefits and limitations
of the examination should be described. They suggest
that it is both unfair and unethical, for example, merely

to tell a patient scheduled for cerebral angiography that he is 'going down to the X-ray department where they will take a few pictures'. This statement omits some unpleasant but highly relevant details concerning the possible hazards of the procedure, which the patient has a right to know before giving his permission.

Hinck and Wagner also point out that in an emergency, examination without consent may be necessary. This applies to unconscious or severe debilitated patients as well as to mentally incompetent or under-age patients. They recommend that in such circumstances a note be made in the patient's chart before the examination indicating: (1) why it is an emergency; (2) why the patient cannot sign his own consent, and (3) that a reasonable effort has been made to contact the next of kin for the purpose of obtaining consent.

The matter of proper information before obtaining consent sometimes becomes the central point in a legal dispute and these authors recommend that after a patient signs a proper consent form, an entry should be made in the clinical notes to the effect that the doctor has described the procedure to the patient and indicated the inherent hazard of serious complication or even fatality. The doctor should add a note that 'to the best of my judgement, the patient understood and accepted the procedure'. This is a wise precaution in view of the increasing number of disputes over alleged inadequate information before consent is obtained. Hinck and Wagner also emphasize the use of broad terms in discussing complications, such as 'mild complication' or 'serious complications'. This was mentioned earlier and is necessary to circumvent a failure to enumerate all the possible complications that may occur.

The foregoing is the 'official' view which is a counsel of perfection often preached by lawyers, the courts and protection and insurance societies. It has been challenged, especially by Robert Allen (1976) who wrote an extremely interesting article subsequent to losing a malpractice case where a fatal outcome occurred after intravenous urography. Allen pointed out that he had performed between 6 and 8000 urograms without ever having a fatal reaction, in a hospital which had been doing urograms for 25 years without any fatalities. When the fatal case came along, it transpired in court that he had not warned the patient of a possible reaction. This was a deliberate policy on his part, as he indicated that it did no good. Allen told the court that if he had told the patient that there was a chance that she might have a reaction and die, it would have distressed her, but after calming her down, he had no doubt that he would have been able to persuade her to have the urogram for the sake of her future health. In other words, even if he had obtained informed consent, and death had occurred, the malpractice suit would still have been brought. Allen also pointed out that the expert witness for the plaintiff was a pathologist who stated that 'It is the standard of medical practice for a radiologist to warn a patient of adverse reactions including death before performing urography'. On cross examination, this witness was unable to give the name of even one radiologist who did this. The case was apparently lost on the matter of 'right to know' and not on the practical issue of whether the obtaining of informed consent would have inhibited the malpractice suit.

Allen points out that the consequence of such legal actions is that as some radiologists are now warning their patients of the possible risks before urography and other radiological procedures, this is making it legally hazardous for the vast majority of radiologists who do not warn their patients. He comments 'We have got into trouble in informed consent by getting legal opinion. What a physician tells a patient before performing urography is part of the practice of medicine. We must make informed consent a medical rather than a legal decision. Do radiologists inform their patients of the risks of urography because they think it is good medicine or do they inform their patients because they think it is good for themselves legally? If you do have a urography reaction, the fact that you warned the patient will in no way prevent a malpractice case from being filed.'

The American College of Radiology has extensively studied the issue of informed consent related to urography and advised all radiologists of the following:

'Our responsibility is to our patients and to do what is best for our patients medically. Informing patients of risks and possible death from urography may not be in the best interest of the patient and some experts feel that it may be dangerous.'

Allen's philosophy has not gone unchallenged and Seymour Ochsner has replied 'Most radiologists would agree with Allen that physicians should establish standards of medical practice. The real problem here is different. Medical standards as we perceive them do not override the legal rights of patients. While I do not pretend to be learned in the law, I have been advised by attornies that a physician's judgement cannot abridge the basic rights of a patient. One of these rights is to be informed about the risks involved in diagnostic procedures. To perform an examination which carried a small but definite risk of fatality is not something that we can do without telling the patient about the small risk—even if we believe it is not "good" medical practice to alarm patients'.

Thus the concept of informed consent is by no means unanimously accepted, but in the small proportion of cases which give rise to legal complications, the absence of proof of any informed consent is very serious stumbling block to a successful defence of the radiologist.

RADIOLOGICAL DIAGNOSIS OF CEREBRAL DEATH

The diagnosis of irreversible arrest of the cerebral circulation has gained in importance in recent years mainly as a result of the advances in transplant surgery. The need for an accurate diagnosis has become urgent.

As the intra-cranial pressure rises the cerebral circulation is progressively reduced eventually leading to irreversible damage to the brain. When the intra-cranial pressure rises to the level of the diastolic blood pressure no blood flow to the brain occurs during cardiac diastole. Venous return is also prevented at this pressure and finally the cerebral circulation ceases when the intra-cranial pressure reaches the systolic blood pressure.

Brain death in patients with cardiac function was defined by a committee at the Harvard Medical School based on the following findings: unreceptiveness and unresponsiveness to intense stimulation, no spontaneous respiration or movement, no reflexes of any kind, and two flat electro-encephalograms at least 24 hours apart in the absence of hypothermia and depressant drugs.

This was followed by the publication of the Conference of Royal Colleges and Faculties of the United Kingdom (October 1976) which laid down specific criteria consisting of the following:

(a) The patient must be deeply comatose.
(b) The patient must be maintained on a ventilator because spontaneous respiration had previously become inadequate or had ceased altogether.
(c) There was no doubt there was irremediable structural brain damage.

Further guidance was given on diagnostic tests for brain death, mainly concerned with the absence of brainstem reflexes.

These criteria were consolidated in a definitive document issued in a Code of Practice on the Removal of Cadaveric Organs for Transplantation issued by the British Department of Health in January 1980.

It has been pointed out by Cantu (1973) that many potential donors are lost during the 24-hour waiting period due to failure to maintain cardiac or renal perfusion.

A number of reports have established the fact that cerebral arteriography provides an accurate and quick method to assess the absence of the cerebral circulation (Rosenklint and Jørgensen, 1974; Greitz et al., 1973; Berquist et al., 1972; Parvey et al., 1976; Bradac et al., 1973). Some authors (Bradac & Simon, 1974) believe that aortic arch angiography is the method of choice. Whatever the method employed the absence of flow in the intra-cerebral arteries or a circulation time exceeding 15 s indicates brain death. The external carotid arteries should have normal flow. Rosenklint and Jørgensen (1974) found in some of their patients differences in perfusion between the supra- and intratentorial circulation. Parvey *et al.* further noted flow through the anterior and posterior communicating arteries with retrograde filling of the cervical portion of the opposite carotid artery and vertebro–basilar system. They also observed compression of the basilar artery against the clivus in some of their patients which they attributed to oedema of the brain stem and cerebellum.

7 Radiological mishaps and malpractice

Although radiologists are not in the same high-risk category of medical negligence and malpractice as orthopaedic and casualty surgeons, plastic surgeons, anaesthetists and general practitioners, they are by no means immune from such allegations, whether ill-founded or otherwise. Many of the incidents arise as a by-product of accident and emergency treatment where the radiologist provides a back-up service to the casualty department. The other fertile source of negligence actions arises from more complex radiological procedures, especially those involving the parenteral introduction of contrast media. Thus allegations of radiological malpractice may arise from commission or omission. Though most of the cases fail to reach actual litigation, due either to a lack of persistence on the part of the complainant or to an obvious lack of supporting evidence, the episodes may provide a worrying and anxious time for the radiologist, which may be drawn out into a period of several years before the matter is finally disposed of. In addition, even though the allegation may be ill-founded, there may be substantial legal costs involved in proving the lack of negligence.

For all these reasons, the services of a medical defence organization in Europe and of adequate insurance cover in the United States are absolutely vital. The radiologist must communicate all relevant facts to his defence society or insurers immediately and make no personal unilateral admissions to the patient or to his legal representatives once it is clear that the patient is set upon litigation. As with all aspects of medical malpractice, a breakdown of the doctor–patient relationship is a potent cause of allegations of negligence, though the radiologist is rarely the primary medical attendant and is more likely to be blamed for more technical reasons than for a failure of clinical rapport.

Indeed, not infrequently he has a vicarious role in malpractice suits, being joined with the clinicians as co-defendant, when he may even never have seen the patient face-to-face, as in alleged faults in reviewing films from a casualty unit.

A number of legal cases have revolved around particular radiological techniques. Though the opportunities for allegations of malpractice are limitless, a series of examples will illustrate many of the risks. The following are taken from American practice.

The first situation concerns failure to take radiographs. If the symptoms presented by the patient are such that no standard practice to order X-ray films exists amongst physicians, it is not negligence if none are taken. For example, in *Hall* v. *Ferry*, a patient complaining of backache was seen by a neurosurgeon and an orthopaedic surgeon, who agreed with her physicians's diagnosis of sciatica. Some time later, she fractured her leg and it was discovered that she had osteomyelitis. It was held that there was no negligence in failing to take radiographs at the time of the first complaint, as it was not standard practice to radiograph the lower limbs in a case of backache.

Where failure to take radiological examinations has not caused damage to the patient, no damages can be recovered. In *Robinson* v. *Gatti*, a doctor saw a patient in the accident department following a traffic accident. No radiography was carried out and a fractured rib and a punctured lung remained undiagnosed until the next day. It was held that mere delay in diagnosis did not constitute damage, since the omission did not cause or contribute to additional suffering.

In *Walden* v. *Jones*, a patient with symptoms including a pain in the back, was diagnosed as a virus infection on other grounds. Paraplegia ensued and some months later another neurosurgeon found a herniated disc on radiological studies. Operation was unsuccessful. The court held that no damages could be recovered, as the patient had submitted no evidence that he would have recovered even if the disc problem had been discovered immediately.

Two cases involving fractures of the hand (*Henry* v. *McCool* and *Thomas* v. *Beckering*) also involved failure to radiograph but it was not proved that this would have made any difference to the progress of the disability.

The general rule in determining whether radiography should be carried out is that of 'due care'. Before a patient can recover for a misdiagnosis as a result of failure to take X-rays, he must show that another physician who was 'duly careful' would have taken radiographs. The patient must also show that radiological examination under the circumstances of his accident or illness would have been standard practice.

Even if the duly careful physician would have submitted the patient for radiological examination and the defendant in a malpractice action did not, the patient must prove more than an error in judgement or diagnosis. He must prove that he suffered damage through failure to take radiographs, apart from the simple delay in the administration of the correct treatment.

Where angiography is concerned, some United States cases are relevant. In *Salgo* v. *the Stanford Board of Trustees*, a patient who became paralysed after an angiogram recovered damages on the grounds that no properly informed consent had been obtained, negligence being present in the failure to furnish any information as to the risk. However, in another case (*Stivers* v. *George Washington University*) a patient's claim for temporary paralysis and speech disorder was unsuccessful as the court rejected her claim that she had not been warned of the risk. In *Bowers* v. *Telmage*, a neurologist who advised parents that a boy with headaches should have an arteriogram, was held negligent because he did not tell them of any potential risk.

In *Ball* v. *Mallinkrodt Chemical Works*, a patient suffered a paraplegia after an aortogram obtained by the injection of acetrizoate sodium (70% solution). Some of the contrast medium had escaped from the aorta and the defence pleaded that this had occurred in spite of the utmost skill and care. The defendant doctor testified that he used this substance instead of another which might have been less toxic, because it permitted better films to be made. The court held that the doctor, in the exercise of his best judgement, had the right to choose those agents recognized by a large number of his colleagues, without being negligent.

In another case, a negligence action was brought because of failure to perform an angiogram. The patient suffered a head injury in hospital and an arteriogram was proposed, but not performed because the patient developed breathing difficulties. At cranio-tomy, no evidence of a haematoma was found, but at autopsy a large epidural haematoma was revealed. The family sued on the grounds that failure to perform the arteriogram was negligence and caused the death of the patient. The court recognized that in a small percentage of cases, an arteriogram has adverse effects and held that the physicians were within the reason-able exercise of their professional judgement to con-clude that this was one of this group (*Solorio* v. *Lampros*). In *Dill* v. *Scuka*, the patient sued because he alleged that the doctor was negligent in not performing a laminectomy to relieve his paralysis after a myelo-gram. Although the patient called expert evidence to suggest that this was a standard practice, the court did not uphold his claim.

Myelography also has produced a few leading cases in the annals of malpractice. Again most of the cases are from the United States. In *Toal* v. *United States*, a veteran successfully claimed damages because of neurological complications caused by failure to remove iophandylate injected into his spine for myelography. A similar case was *Mathis* v. *Hejna*, where a patient developed arachnoiditis as a result of failure to remove the iophandylate injection.

In *Ciccarone* v. *United States*, a patient claimed negligence due to an idiosyncratic reaction or allergy to the contrast medium used in a myelogram, maintain-ing that the radiologist should have performed sensiti-vity tests prior to performing the procedure. The court accepted expert testimony that no such test was available.

In *Walden* v. *Jones*, a patient with a paraplegia was suspected of having a spinal tumour. A myelogram revealed no tumour and the films were not examined for any other abnormality. At a later date, another doctor discovered a herniated disc, but the delay allegedly made the condition untreatable. The patient claimed a more careful inspection of the X-ray films would have revealed the disc lesion and that prompt surgery would have alleviated his paralysis. The court declined to accept that earlier diagnosis would have affected the outcome.

In *Berkey* v. *Anderson*, a patient developed foot-drop after a myelogram. The patient claimed that neither his physician nor a neurologist had given him any idea of what the procedure entailed much less what risks were involved.

In *Hale* v. *Henninger*, a myelogram revealed a herniated disc. A laminectomy was performed immediately after the myelogram, but the patient became paralysed. He sued both the radiologist and the surgeon.

Legal aspects of mammography. Gershon-Cohen (1970) has pointed out the legal implications of mammography. The radiologist might be expected to make a correct diagnosis of carcinoma in more than 85% of patients submitted to mammography, which is almost as accurate as biopsy diagnosis.

It is recommended that the radiologist should always familiarize himself with the findings of the referring physician or surgeon, concerning the findings of physical examination and what the patient has been told. The radiologist should then make his own physical examination and if any palpable lesion is found, it is as well to mark this area by fixing a minute lead shot with adhesive tape so that it might be identified on films.

He should verify the accuracy of the projections, where again the lead shot can be of considerable assistance.

Where the clinical and radiological findings are similar, the accuracy of diagnosis reaches 90% or more. If there is a difference, then a biopsy would appear to be the only proper course to follow.

If the radiologist discovers a lesion on the mammograms such as micro-calcification it is important to radiograph the biopsy specimen to ascertain whether the lesion in question has been removed. Furthermore identifying the exact position of the abnormality can be vital to the pathologist if the correct diagnosis is to be made. Close collaboration between surgeons, radiologists and pathologists will avoid mistakes such as mastectomy for benign disease.

The following examples are taken—with due acknowledgment—from the informative and salutary Annual Reports issued by the Medical Defence Union and the Medical Protection Society in Britain.

The summaries are representative of the difficulties in which radiologists may find themselves. They are by no means exhaustive—indeed, a famous aphorism of a High Court judge in a negligence case was that 'The categories of negligence are never closed'. Every new radiological technique presents a new opportunity for something to go wrong, but human error is still far more common than failure of the 'hardware'.

A 60-year-old actor underwent a barium enema which appeared to proceed normally, no leak from the rectum being detected on screening or on films. Later the same day the patient returned to hospital when radiographs revealed that barium had entered the pelvic tissues, indicating a perforation. A temporary colostomy was performed. The patient sued, claiming that he had suffered extreme discomfort during the procedure and that a self-retaining catheter should not have been used. He also claimed loss of earnings as an actor-writer. Expert advice indicated that perforation of the colon is a rare but well recognized hazard in barium enemas, particularly when used to investigate ulcerative colitis. Nevertheless, the films taken after the examination clearly showed an extravazation of barium, which should have been recognized and reported by the radiologist. The patient's claim was successful.

A yachtsman was struck in the face by a rope, which smashed his spectacles. He attended a casualty department complaining of glass in his eye, but the casualty officer did not detect a foreign body. He prescribed antibiotics, but took no X-ray. He was seen by another doctor at a later stage, when panophthalmitis was present. The patient claimed damages and was successful.

Though it is often stated that glass is almost invariably radio-opaque, this does not necessarily apply to glass fragments in the orbit particularly if these are small.

Foreign bodies in the eye regularly give rise to claims for negligence and omission to take radiographs is frequently part of the plaintiff's case. A young workman felt something enter his eye while using a pneumatic drill and was seen by hospital ophthalmic surgeons. A foreign body was embedded in the cornea and was removed. Radiological examination was not carried out as it was thought that the injury had been adequately treated. Nine months later the patient came back with conjunctivitis and episcleral infection. The eye improved on steroids, but more than a year later radiology revealed an intra-ocular foreign body which was removed at operation. A cataract developed and a second operation was necessary to remove the lens. The patient made a successful claim for negligence in the delayed diagnosis of the intra-ocular foreign body.

Foreign bodies, especially glass, give rise to many claims where failure to X-ray is the leading matter. A general practitioner took his patient to a cottage hospital after a hand injury from glass and finding no foreign body on clinical examination, sutured the wound. There were no untoward results for about a year, when pain and difficulty in flexing the index finger caused further investigation and X-ray revealed a piece of glass in the hand. Negligence was alleged, but it was not pursued after it was pointed out to the claimant that it is not always possible or desirable to X-ray every minor injury.

A 10-year-old boy was brought to hospital with a history of having been hit on the head with the handle of a garden rake. There was a laceration of the scalp but a skull X-ray viewed by the casualty officer was, in his opinion, normal. The films were also shown to a surgical registrar who also considered that there was no evidence of a fracture. The boy was discharged home, but was re-admitted next day and died on transfer to a neurosurgical unit. At the inquest, autopsy photographs indicated that there was a 3-in. fracture of the skull which the pathologist said should have been palpable through the scalp. The coroner stated that there had been a misreading of the X-ray plates and the boy's father requested an investigation by the Area Health Authority.

A doctor, though not on duty, was asked to see a little girl with pain in her arm following a fall. The doctor examined the X-ray films and could see no obvious bone injury, but suspected a displacement of the medial epiconyle. A claim for negligence in failing to diagnose was made, but this was repudiated and was not pursued.

A footballer was admitted to hospital with a lacerated leg and a fractured tibia and fibula. Suturing and traction were carried out. Two days later, X-rays were taken, but gas shadows were not acted upon by either consultant surgeon nor radiologist who saw the films. It was another two days before gas gangrene was diagnosed from obvious clinical signs and penicillin therapy begun. Eventually, below-knee amputation had to be performed. Two years later, an action was brought for negligence in not properly cleaning the wound, failing at first viewing to diagnos gas gangrene which should have been seen on the radiographs. The claim was settled for £26 000.

A lady attended a casualty unit after a road accident, having sustained injury to her hip and lacerated upper arm. The casualty officer had the relevant areas X-rayed and was satisfied that there was no bony injury. Ten days later, the lady went to another hospital complaining of pain in the arm and a large piece of metal was removed from the arm wound. This was visible on the first X-rays, but was assumed to be an artefact by the casualty officer. The claim was settled for a modest amount. At the hospital, it was the practice for a radiologist to review only skull and chest films, the remainder being reported solely by the casualty officers.

In a parallel case, a fractured femur was missed after radiography when the film was seen by the casualty officer. The routine review report by a radiologist arrived, one week later, by which time the patient was admitted moribund from chest infection, and the relatives brought an action for negligence.

A 30-year-old man attended his general practitioner on nine occasions with an unresolved chest infection. On a subsequent visit, he saw a locum doctor who ordered a chest X-ray, but left the practice before the report arrived, which suggested active tuberculosis. The report was not seen by either of the two regular practitioners and a secretary mis-filed it between two envelopes in a filing cabinet, where it remained for six months. The patient attended fourteen times in the interval, his symptoms worsening until he had to be admitted to hospital eight months after the X-ray. A successful action was brought against the practice and a settlement in excess of £36 000 obtained.

A middle-aged woman attended a casualty department after injuring her arm in a fall. A locum consultant saw her and found a painful arm with no clinical signs of fracture. He did not order an X-ray. Five weeks later, there was muscle wasting and restriction of movement and an orthopaedic surgeon discovered a sub-coracoid dislocation of the humerus. Extensive joint changes ensued with permanent disfigurement and limitation of movement. An action for negligence in not X-raying the original injury was settled for costs and damages of £4500.

The missed scaphoid fracture is a regular source of mishap. A victim of a car accident attended hospital with hand injuries which were sutured. He was told to return next day for X-rays, when he was seen by another doctor who ordered 'wrist X-rays' which were reported as 'no bony injury'.

For five months he consulted his G.P. with pain and eventually made a private visit to an orthopaedic surgeon who discovered bilateral scaphoid fractures with wide displacement. The patient sued, confining his claim to the medical costs only and the action was settled.

If a scaphoid fracture is remotely suspected, then special views must be requested, rather than a vague 'Please X-ray, query fracture'.

A girl lacerated her leg on a glass door at school. This

was sutured at a casualty department, but sixteen months later, she was referred by her family doctor for severe pain in the thigh. Radiography revealed a piece of glass clearly visible in the healed wound. A claim for negligence was settled. The casualty officer did not have X-rays because he thought that glass was not radio-opaque, though in fact most glass, being composed of sodium or potassium silicate casts recognizable shadows even when superimposed on bone.

Another man with multiple lacerations of his arm from a broken window was sutured by a casualty officer. Six weeks later, pain and restriction of movement caused him to return, when radiography revealed four foreign bodies in his arm. Three pieces of glass were removed, but the patient was told that the fourth could not be found. He instituted a successful claim for damages. One of the doctors concerned said on hearing of the claim that 'glass seldom if ever shows up on X-rays' though this statement is patently incorrect.

A 39-year-old man became paraplegic after renal angiography for the investigation of his hypertension. A claim was made that the contrast medium was over-concentrated and in excessive quantity. Though the type of medium was held to be correct, it was admitted that the concentration was excessive for renal angiography. The claim was settled for £125 000 and £10 000 costs.

A young man referred for radiology for back pain, was reported by the radiologist to have no significant abnormality, even though in retrospect the films showed a destroyed disc and probably vertebral body destruction. The general practitioner had previously recorded 'TB is high on the list? tuberculosis?'. The negative report was filed, but a week later dramatic deterioration occurred. Myelography and neurosurgery was necessary, revealing a tuberculous spinal abscess. The patient sued for negligence and delayed diagnosis and was awarded £20 000.

A boy of 17 suffered a fractured neck of the femur in a road accident, reported by a radiologist as being intertrochanteric. It was pinned and the patient eventually discharged. Months later, solicitors requested an opinion on the likelihood of osteoarthritic changes and the request was dealt with by a new registrar. He was of the opinion that as it was intertrochanteric fracture, the joint capsule was not damaged so the prognosis was good.

The patient settled his claim with an insurance company in respect of the accident, but two years later, avascular necrosis of the head of the femur developed. As no claim could be now made against the insurers, the patient sought to recover the difference from the doctors in view of their incorrect prognosis. It was then found that the radiologist was in error and that the fracture was intra-capsular, this giving a much worse risk of developing joint changes. A settlement in excess of £20 000 including costs was made.

A 19-year-old man injured his wrist in a traffic accident and attended a casualty department where radiology revealed a scaphoid fracture. However, the inexperienced casualty officer failed to notice the lesions, which was picked up on review by a radiologist next day. The radiologist reported this to the casualty consultant, who wrote an instruction on the casualty card for the patient to attend the next fracture clinic and a notification was posted to the patient. However, he never came and later claimed that he had never received the request. It was six weeks before continuing pain sent the patient to an orthopaedic surgeon. A claim for £23 000 was made against the driver of the other vehicle and the health authority.

A locum radiologist, working with unfamiliar apparatus was to screen an elderly lady having a barium enema. As there was a male radiographer present, an unqualified female nurse was told to insert a catheter in the rectum, following which the radiologist allowed the barium to run in. He rapidly saw from the screening that something was amiss and stopped the barium flow, but the woman died within two minutes. It was found that the catheter had been inserted in the vagina by mistake and death was due to rupture of the vagina due to the introduction of barium under pressure.

A house officer, deputizing for a casualty officer, attended a patient who had injured his hip in a road accident. The hip was X-rayed and the poor quality films were regarded as normal by the house officer. The patient was discharged, but the following day a radiologist reviewed the films and diagnosed a fractured neck of the femur. His report was filed with the patient's records, but was never brought to the attention of the house surgeon or casualty officer. A few weeks later the patient attended another hospital, where the fractured femur was diagnosed. The delay in treating the fracture had unfortunate consequences and the patient's claim for damages was settled out of court.

The young son of the friend of a surgeon was hit in the elbow by an airgun pellet. The surgeon decided to remove the pellet in theatre under direct X-ray screening, though in fact this was unsuccessful in locating the pellet. Five days later the arm became red and later the skin broke down due to an X-ray burn, which developed into a chronic ulcer. Prolonged treatment and plastic surgery was required. In addition, ten days after the operation, the surgeon developed milder X-ray burns to three of his fingers which had been involved in the operative area. This resolved satisfactorily, but scarring and limitation of movement of the elbow of the patient led to a successful claim of £3000.

A healthy man was admitted to hospital for investigation of suspected pulmonary tuberculosis, though in fact his chest film had been wrongly labelled and confused with another at the chest clinic. A subsequent X-ray was normal and the patient was discharged, but he claimed against the physician, the claim including damages accruing to his wife who had alleged that she had been so distressed at the possibility of her husband having tuberculosis that she forgot to take 'the Pill' and became pregnant. The claim was unsuccessful.

A radiologist was using apparatus which was not shockproof and a patient sustained a burn on the back with damage to her clothing due to a spark between the X-ray tube and the metal chair upon which she was sitting. No real defence could be raised, though the quantum of damages was reduced from that claimed by the patient.

A locum general practitioner mistakenly referred a pregnant woman for an intravenous pyelogram. The mistake probably arose by having two record cards on his desk at the same time. The referral form was completed in the name of the pregnant woman. The same doctor was acting as radiologist in the local hospital and actually gave the intravenous injection, failing to recognize the woman as the one he had seen previously to confirm her pregnancy. As a result, eight films were taken of the lower abdominal and pelvic region of the woman who was thirteen weeks pregnant. Though she was told that there was a very small chance of fetal damage, she became greatly distressed and elected to have the pregnancy terminated.

After a stripping operation for varicose veins, a swab was reported missing. The surgeon instructed his house officer to have the patient X-rayed, but unfortunately the films were only taken of the groin area. A few weeks later, the swab was removed at another hospital from the patient's left leg, below the area previously radiographed. The patient sued and was successful.

A radiologist advised screening of a patient, involving the introduction of barium paste into the pharynx. The introduction was carried out by a radiographer, but the cork and foil sealing-pad from inside the cap of the barium tube was stuck to the nozzle of the tube and was introduced into the pharynx. This became lodged in the upper oesophagus and had to be removed under general anaesthesia. A claim was made against the radiologist because he was vicariously liable for the radiographer. In this case, the claim was resisted on the grounds that the manufacturers of the tube were liable and the claim was settled by them with a small contribution on behalf of the doctor.

An eye injury sustained by a man at work was referred to the accident department of a hospital, where a corneal abrasion was diagnosed and a radiograph of the orbit taken. Two days later another doctor saw the patient again, when the abrasion had healed and again an X-ray was not taken. Two days later, the patient returned to the ophthalmic clinic because of a congested eye and here radiology revealed a metallic fragment embedded in the eye. Infection followed and the eye was eviscerated. The patient sued for negligence and the claim was settled for £1200.

Injuries to the wrist are common and a missed scaphoid fracture is also common. Radiographic abnormalities may be delayed for several weeks after the injury and courts expect even newly qualified doctors to be aware of this. As an example, a young woman admitted to a maternity hospital fell in the ward bathroom and injured her wrist. An X-ray revealed no fracture but the patient continued to complain of pain in the wrist and ten months later was seen by another doctor who ordered a radiograph which revealed a fracture of the scaphoid. A claim was settled out of court.

An aortic arch angiogram was carried out to investigate a suspected carotid artery embolus in a 57-year-old man. The experienced senior registrar in radiology attempted a femoral puncture, but this proved impossible because of local atheroma and successful catheterization was carried out via an axillary artery. When a test injection was made to check the position of the catheter, the patient complained of pain at the puncture site. Radiographic appearances were satisfactory, the investigation was completed and the catheter was withdrawn. That evening the patient developed weakness of the hand muscles with impairment of sensation in the fingers. This gradually improved and was thought to be a lesion of the brachial plexus with involvement of the muscles innervated by the median and ulnar nerves, a sequel of arch angiograms which is recorded in the literature. Three years later, the patient's lawyers alleged almost total paralysis of the small muscles of the right hand with other weakness and loss of sensation. Expert opinion was that the patient would improve slowly and that there was nothing to suggest that the doctor had been negligent in carrying out the angiogram. The case eventually came to the High Court, but no radiologist was called to give evidence on the plaintiff's behalf and the case was dismissed after a trial lasting one week.

8 Some medico-legal considerations in the radiology of trauma: healing of fractures

HEAD INJURIES

There is considerable controversy regarding the value of skull radiography in trauma. The mere presence of a skull fracture unless it involves a sinus or is depressed is not of importance. Damage to the intra-cranial contents can occur without a skull fracture and this can only be assessed by a careful clinical examination. However, Ulin *et al.* (1955) found a significantly higher mortality in patients with cerebral injuries and skull fracture than in those with cerebral injury without skull fractures. On the other hand, Bell and Loop (1971) expressed considerable doubt regarding the value of skull radiographs in trauma and the clinical significance of a skull fracture. Most authors are agreed that skull radiography is mandatory to localize a foreign body and to detect depressed or compound fractures.

In many centres the presence or absence of a skull fracture determines whether patients are admitted to hospital for observation. It could be argued that a proportion of such patients are admitted unnecessarily but on the other hand a greater proportion are sent home who might otherwise have been admitted to hospital. Routine views of the skull in trauma should include postero–anterior, horizontal-lateral and Towne's projection. Other projections such as tangential views in possible depressed fractures and tomograms in injuries to the petrous bones may be required.

It may be difficult to differentiate linear fractures from suture lines or vascular grooves. Fractures are usually unilateral, often cross the lines of sutures or vessels, and are generally more sharply defined than the margins of sutures or vessels. Furthermore when they change direction this occurs with a sharp angulation.

Depressed fragments produce areas of increased density (Fig. 8.1) due to overlapping areas of bone. Tangential radiographs are of particular importance to assess the degree of compression.

Fractures of the base of the skull are difficult to demonstrate. Those involving the middle fossa usually extend into the sphenoid sinus. In such cases the lateral radiograph with a horizontal beam often shows an air-fluid level within the sphenoidal sinus. The presence of an intra-cranial aerocele will also be shown with this projection.

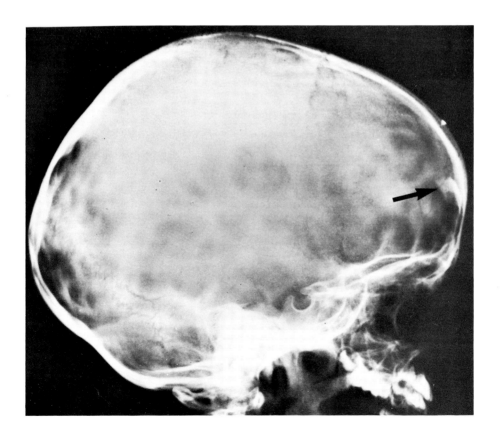

Fig. 8.1. Depressed fracture of the skull showing increased density at the fracture site due to overlap of the skull fragments.

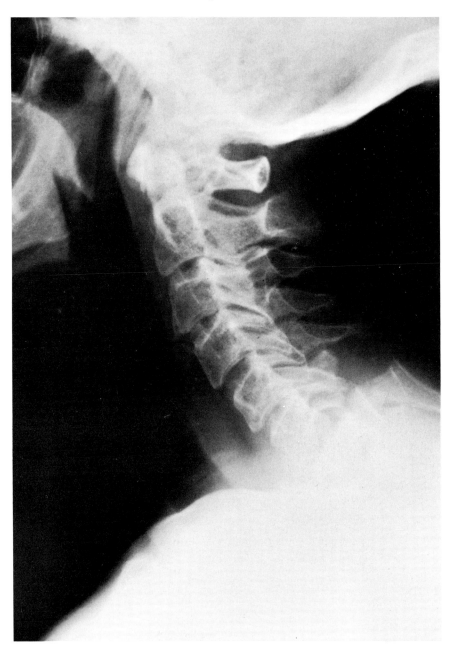

Fig. 8.2. Fracture of the body of
the 7th cervical vertebra with
loss of alignment. Difficult to
see on original radiograph.

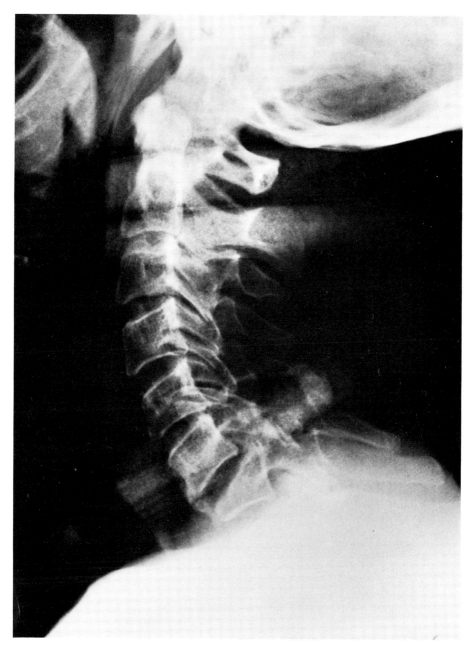

Fig. 8.2b. Subsequent
radiograph showing fracture of
the body of the seventh cervical
vertebra.

Radiology in other areas

It is of great importance in all cases of trauma that radiographs at right angles should always be obtained. It is common experience for a significant fracture only to be revealed on one projection. In the long bones the nearest joint to the site of injury must always be included on the radiograph.

The spine

In patients with injury to the cervical spine it is frequently extremely difficult to obtain a lateral radiograph which includes all seven cervical vertebrae. The author has witnessed two patients in whom inadequate radiography has resulted in misleading reports so that patients with damage to the lower cervical spine were sent home only to return with severe neurological damage. In such cases if radiographs demonstrating all seven cervical vertebrae are impossible to obtain, tomography must be performed (Fig. 8.2).

The severity of injury to the spine may produce associated haemorrhage or oedema so that the pre-vertebral or para-vertebral soft tissue shadows may be increased. This on occasion may be a most important sign of trauma. One recent case of medico-legal importance concerned a young woman who had been involved in a traffic accident following which she was admitted to hospital with concussion. An initial radiograph of the dorsal spine (Fig. 8.3) showed slight lateral wedging of the lower dorsal vertebra. These were considered to be congenital in origin and not the result of injury. However the presence of a para-vertebral haematoma had not been recognized. This indicated severe trauma and substantial damages were awarded.

The limbs

Posterior dislocation of the shoulder, though rare (4%) is of particular importance because it is not recognized in a significant number of cases. The reason for the

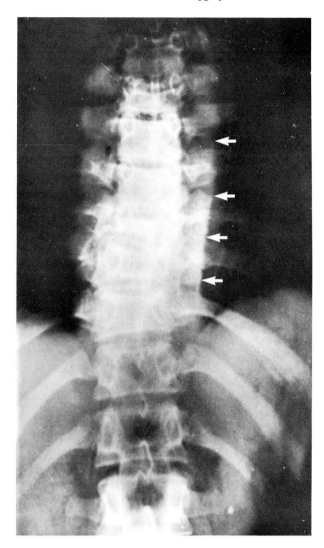

Fig. 8.3. Lateral wedging of the lower dorsal vertebra with a large para-vertebral haematoma.

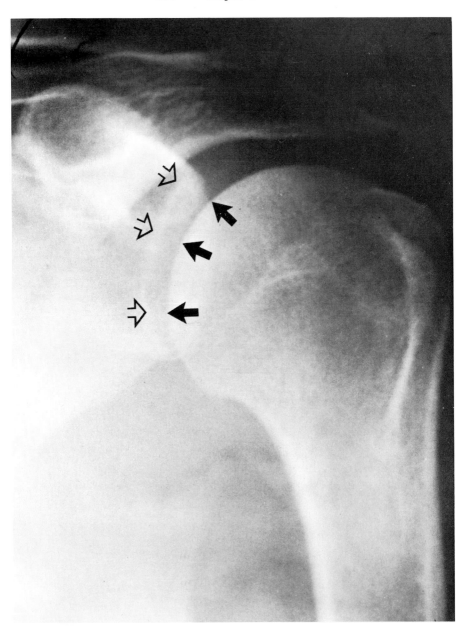

Fig. 8.4. (a) Antero–posterior radiograph of normal shoulder joint.

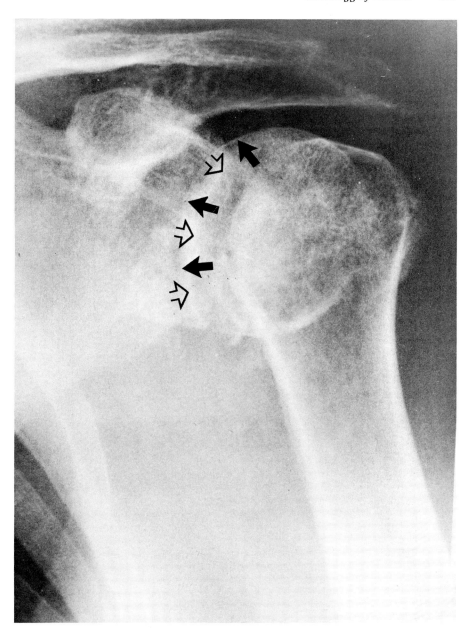

Fig. 8.4. (b) Fracture posterior
dislocation of the shoulder
joint. Note the humeral head
overlapping the margin of the
glenoid, rotation of the humeral
head and loss of parallelism
between the humeral head and
glenoid margin

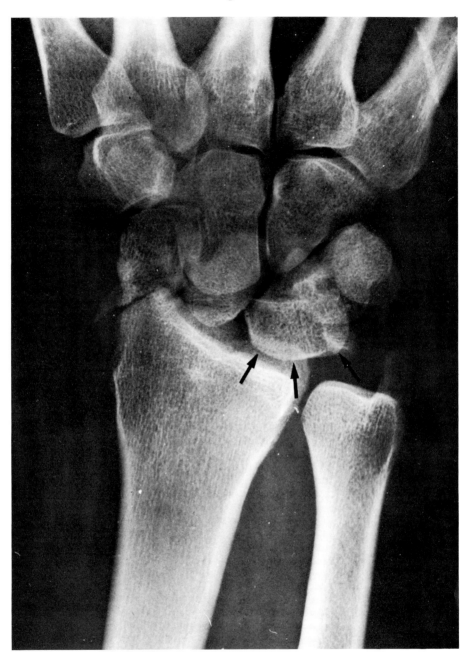

Fig. 8.5. (a) Dislocation of the
lunate. The normal relationship
between the lunate and
capitate is lost.
Antero–posterior projection

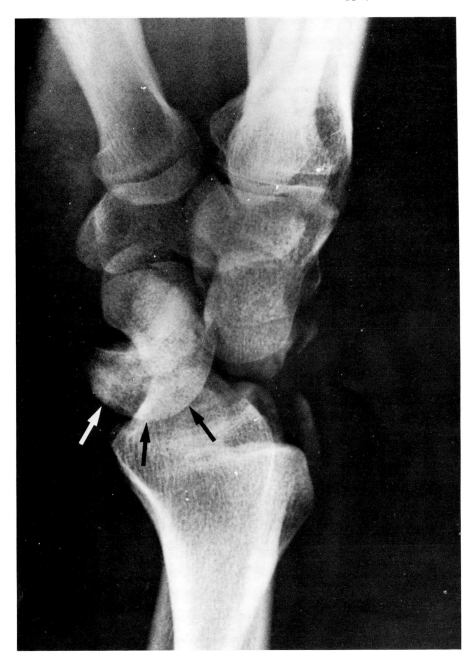

Fig. 8.5. (b) Lateral projection.

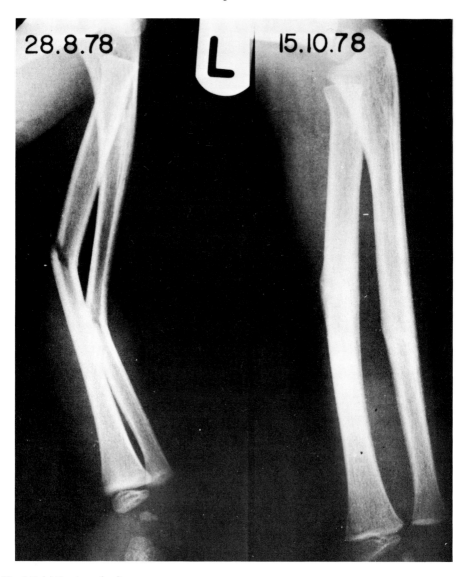

Fig. 8.6. (a) Fracture of radius and ulna showing complete healing in 7 weeks.

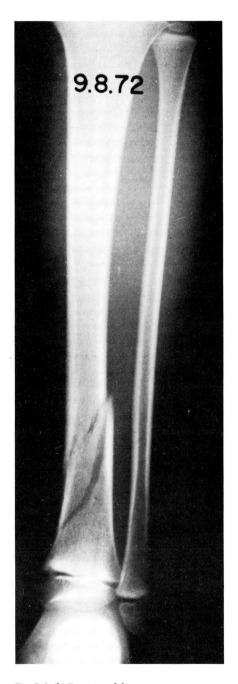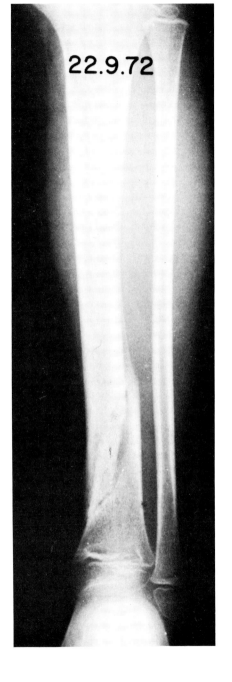

Fig. 8.6. (b) Fracture of the tibia. After almost 7 weeks the fracture line is still clearly visible and very little callus has formed.

failure in diagnosis arises because the radiograph in the antero–posterior projection appears remarkably normal. However, there is often superimposition of the humeral head upon the glenoid fossa and the space between the humeral head and the anterior margins of the glenoid fossa is widened. In addition there may be loss of parallelism between the humeral head and the glenoid fossa and the marked internal rotation of the humerus results in the head and neck shown 'end on'. (Fig. 8.4). An axial view readily defines a posterior dislocation and again emphasizes the importance of radiographs at right angles. In the elbow joint soft tissue abnormalities are of considerable importance, as they may be the only obvious abnormality. Injuries of the elbow joint that produce intra-articular haemorrhage displace the extra-capsular fat both anteriorly and posteriorly. The so-called 'fat pad' sign is strongly suggestive of intra-articular trauma.

In cases where injury to the forearm has produced a fracture of the ulna with anterior or posterior angulation a radiograph of the elbow joint should always be obtained because of the association with dislocation of the proximal radius (Monteggia fracture).

Lunate and peri-lunate dislocations in the wrist joint again emphasize the necessity for radiographs in two planes. In lunate dislocation the lunate is dislocated anteriorly where the capitate moves proximally near the distal radius. In the antero–posterior projection portions of lunate and scaphoid bones are superimposed. The lateral view shows forward dislocation of the lunate (Fig. 8.5). In peri-lunate dislocation the lunate retains its normal relationship with the distal ulna whereas the remainder of the carpal bones are dislocated dorsally. In the antero–posterior projection the capitate is superimposed on the lunate.

The healing of fractures

Fracture healing is one of the bodies' reactions to trauma; in the long bones non-union is always pathological provided the bone ends are in contact and have been adequately immobilized. However, immobilization is not necessary for the healing of rib fractures, the upper end of the humerus or in the pelvis where callus formation is normally abundant. In the femur and tibia, however, callus formation is scant and immobilization is necessary for healing to occur.

It would be of great value in forensic work if radiology could give an accurate assessment of the date of fractures. Non-union normally occurs and is not a pathological process in fractures of the skull in adults. In children skull fractures usually heal in 6–8 months. The dating of such fractures is therefore impossible.

The amount of callus shown on a radiograph not only varies according to the site but varies from patient to patient. Exuberant callus is a feature of patients on steroids and with Cushing's syndrome and hyperplastic callus is seen in some patients with osteogenesis imperfecta. Diminished callus would be expected in patients with osteoporosis, osteomalacia or rickets.

Callus formation is not usually evident radiologically before ten days and gradually increases. There is considerable variation within the normal range and assessment of the date of a fracture can never be precise. Similarly as fractures heal at different rates in different bones it may be difficult to determine whether the fractures have all occurred at the same time. The variation in healing of fractures and the amount of callus formed is shown in (Fig. 8.6). The fracture of the tibia shows only minimal healing after seven weeks whereas the forearm bones have completely united within a similar time span.

References

ADAMS P.C., STRAND R.D., BRESNAN M.J. & LUCKY A.W. (1974) Kinky Hair Syndrome: serial study of radiological findings with emphasis on the similarity to the Battered Child Syndrome. *Radiology*, **112**, 401–7.

AKESTER J. (1979) Disappearing dycal. *British Dental Journal*, **146**, 369.

ALLEN R.W. (1976) Informed consent. A medical decision. *Radiology*, **119**, 232–4.

ASHERSON N. (1965) *Identification by frontal sinus prints: a forensic medicine pilot survey.* H. K. Lewis & Co., London.

ATKINSON A.B. & KELLETT R.J. (1974) Value of intravenous urography in investigating hypertension. *Journal of the Royal College of Physicians of London*, **8**, 175.

BELL S. & LOOP J.W. (1971) The utility and futility of radiographic skull examination for trauma. *The New England Journal of Medicine*, 284–6.

BERGEN R.P. (1974) Ownership of X-ray films. *Journal of the American Medical Association*, **230**, 1454.

BERQUIST E. & BERGSTRÖM K. (1972) Angiography in cerebral death. *Acta Radiologica* (Stockh.), **12**, 283–8.

BONGIOVI J.J. & LOGOSSO R.D. (1969) Pancreatic pseudocyst occurring in the Battered Child Syndrome. *Journal of Pediatric Surgery*, **4**, 2 (April), 220–6.

BONILLA-SANTIAGO J. & FILL W.L. (1978) Sand aspiration in drowning and near drowning. *Radiology*, **128**, 301–2.

BOSTRÖM K., (1973) Identification from Roentgenograms of *Sinus Frontalis* and *Sella Turcica*. *Proceedings 5th meeting Scandinavian Society of Forensic Medicine*, 309–10.

BOWEN D.A.L. (1966) Role of radiology and identification of foreign bodies at post-mortem examination. *Journal of Forensic Science Society*, **6**, 28.

BOYSEN B.E. (1975) Chylous ascites. Manifestation of the Battered Child syndrome. *American Journal Diseases of Childhood*, **129**, 1338.

BRADAC G.B. & SIMON R.S. (1974) Angiography in brain death. *Neuroradiology*, **7**, 105–8.

BRILL P.W., EWING M.L. & DUNN A.A. (1973) The value of routine chest radiography in children and adolescents. *Pediatrics*, **52**, 125.

BROADBENT B.H. (1937) The face of the normal child. *Angle Orthodontist*, **7**, 183–208.

BROWN R.F. (1976) Prepared remarks for the 10 October 1976 A.C.R. Press Conference. See also *Wall Street Journal*, 21 October 1976.

BROWN R.F., SHAVER J.W. & LAMEL D.A. (1976) *A concept and proposal concerning the radiation exposure of women.* University of California. RHSEP Publication No. 874.

BROWN T.C. (1950) Medical Identification in the Noronic disaster. *Fingerprint and Identification Magazine*, **6** (32), 3–14.

BROWN T.C., DELANEY R.J. & ROBINSON W.L. (1952) Medical identification in the Noronic disaster. *Journal of the American Medical Association*, **148**, 621–7.

CAFFEY J. (1946) Multiple fractures in the long bones in infants suffering from chronic subdural hematoma. *American Journal of Roentgenology*, **56**, 163.

CAFFEY J. (1950) *Pediatric X-ray diagnosis*, 2nd ed., p. 79. Yearbook Publishers, Chicago.

CAFFEY J. (1972) Parent-infant traumatic stress syndrome: (Caffey–Kempe Syndrome), (Battered Babe Syndrome). First Annual Neuhauser Presidential Address of Society for Pediatric Radiology. *American Journal of Roentgenology, Radiology, Therapy & Nuclear Medicine*, **114**, 217–29.

CAFFEY J. (1974) The Whiplash Shaken Infant Syndrome: Manual shaking by the extremities with whiplash-induced intracranial and intraocular bleedings, linked with residual permanent brain damage and mental retardation. *Pediatrics*, **54** (4), 396–403.

CAMERON J.M. & MANT A.K. (1972) Fatal subarachnoid haemorrhage associated with cervical trauma. *Medicine Science & Law*, **12**, 66–70.

CAMERON J.M., JOHNSON H.R.M. & CAMPS F.E. (1966) *Medicine, Science and Law*, **6** (1), 2–21.

CAMERON J.M. & SIMS B.G. (1974) In: *Forensic Dentistry* p. 89. Churchill Livingstone, Edinburgh & London.

CAMPS F.E. (1969) Injuries sustained by children from violence. In: *Recent Advances in Forensic Pathology*, (ed. F. E. Camps), p. 129. Churchill, London.

CANTU R.C. (1973) Brain death as determined by cerebral arteriography. *The Lancet*, **i**, 1391–2.

CARMICHAEL J.H.E. & BERRY R.J. (1976) Diagnostic X-rays in late pregnancy and in the neonate. *Lancet*, **i**, 351.

CARMICHAEL J.H.E. & WARRICK C.K. (1978) Radiology now. The ten day rule—principles and practice. *The British Journal of Radiology*, **51**, 843.

CHEEVERS L.S. & ASCENCIO R. (1977) Identification by skull superimposition. *International Journal of Forensic Dentistry*, **4**, 14–16.

CONTOSTAVLOS D.L. (1971) Massive subarachnoid haemorrhage due to laceration of the vertebral artery associated with fracture of the transverse process of the atlas. *Journal Forensic Science*, **16**, 40–56.

COOKE B.E.D. (1957) Benign fibro-osseous enlargements of the jaws. *British Dental Journal*, **102**, 1–14.

CORNWELL W.S. (1956) Radiography and photography in problems of identification. *Medicine Radiography and Photography*, **32** (1), 34.

CULBERT W.L. & LAW F.M. (1927) Identification by comparison of roentgenograms, of nasal accessory sinuses and mastoid processes. *Journal of the American Dental Association*, **88**, 1634–6.

DEMIRJIAN A., GOLDSTEIN, H. & TANNER J.M. (1973) A new system of dental age assessment. *Human Biology*, **45**, 211–27.

DEVORE D.T. (1977) Radiology and photography in forensic dentistry. *Dental Clinics of North America*, **21**, 69–83.

D.H.S.S. (1979) *The Removal of Cadaveric Organs for Transplantation—A Code of Practice*. Department of Health, London.

DRENNAN M.R. & KEEN J.A. (1953) In: *Identity in Medical Jurisprudence* (ed. I. Gordon, R. Turner and T. W. Price), 3rd ed. p. 336–72. Churchill Livingstone, Edinburgh.

DUTRA F.R. (1944) Identification of a person and estimation of the cause of death from skeletal remains. *Archives of Pathology*, **38**, 339.

EVERSOLE L.R., SABES W.R. & ROVIN S. (1972) Fibrous displasia: a nosologic problem in the diagnosis of fibrio-osseous lesions of the law. *Journal of Oral Pathology*, **1**, 189–220.

FASTLICHT S. (1948) Tooth mutilations in pre-columbian Mexico. *Journal of the American Dental Association*, **36**, 315–23.

FATTEH A.V. & MANN G.T. (1969) The role of radiology in forensic pathology. *Medical Science and Law*, **9**, 27.

FISER R.H., KAPLAN J. & HOLDER J.C. (1972) Congenital syphilis mimicking the Battered Child Syndrome—How does one tell them apart? *Clinical Pediatrics (Phila)*, **11** (5), 305–7.

FLECKER H. (1932) Roentgenographic observations of the human skeleton prior to birth. *Medical Journal of Australia*, **19**, 640–3.

FLECKER H. (1932/33) Roentgenographic observations of the times of appearance of the epiphyses and their fusion with the diaphyses. *JA*, **67**, 118–64.

FLECKER H. (1942) Time of appearance and fusion of ossification centres as observed by roentgenographic methods. *American Journal Roentgenology and Radiographic Therapy*, **47** (1), 97–159.

FONTANA V.J. (1971) *The Maltreated Child*, 2nd ed., p. 5–21. Charles C. Thomas, Springfield, Ill.

FRANCIS C.C., WERLE P.P. & BEHM A. (1939) The appearance of centers of ossification from birth to five years. *American Journal Physiology Anthropology*, **24**, 273–99.

FRANCIS C.C. (1951) The appearances of centres of ossification in human pelvis before birth. *American Journal Roentgenology*, **65**, 778–83.

FRIMANN-DAHL J. (1960) *Roentgen Examinations in Acute Abdominal Diseases*. Charles C. Thomas, Springfield, Ill.

FRYKHOLM K.O., HENRIKSON C.O. & FRYKHOLM A. (1973) The use of iodine-125 X-ray unit at the site of the aeroplane disaster at Dubai. *International Journal of Forensic Dentistry*, **1**, 3–6.

FULLER R.H. (1963) The clinical pathology of human near-drowning. *Proceedings of the Royal Society of Medicine*, **56**, 33–8.

FURNESS J. (1976) Positive dental identification. *International Journal of Forensic Dentistry*, **3**, 2–5.

FURUHATA & YAMAMOTO (1967) *Forensic Odontology*, Springfield Ill: Thomas.

GARN S.M., LEWIS A.B & POLACHECK D.L. (1959) Variability of tooth formation. *Journal of Dental Research*, **38**, 135–48.

GEE D.J. (1975) Radiology in Forensic Pathology. *Radiography*, XL1, 485, 109–14.

GERSHON-COHEN J. (1970) Medical and Legal Implications of Mammography. *Surgery, Gynaecology and Obstetrics*, Feb., 347–8.

GIL D.G. (1969) Physical abuse of children; findings and implications of nationwide survey. *Pediatrics, Supplement*, **44**, 857.

GLAISTER & BRASH (1937) *Medico-legal Aspects of the Ruxton Case* (the dental evidence of identification) Edinburgh: Livingstone.

GLAUSER F.L. & SMITH W.R. (1975) Pulmonary interstitial fibrosis following near-drowning and exposure to short-term high oxygen concentrations. *Chest*, **68**, 373.

GORDON I.R.S. & ROSS F.G.M. (1977) *Diagnostic Radiology in Paediatrics*, p. 340. Butterworths, London.

GORELICK L. (1975) Near eastern cylinder seals studied with dental radiography. *Dental Radiography and Photography*, **48**, 17–21.

GORNALL P., AHMED S., JOLLEYS A. & COHEN S.J. (1972) Intra-abdominal injuries in the Battered Baby Syndrome. *Archives of Disease in Childhood*, **47**, 211.

GRAHAM S., LEVIN M.L., LILIENFIELD A.M., SCHUMAN I., GIBSON R., DOWD J.E. & HEMPELMANN L. (1966) Pre-conception and post-natal irradiation as related to leukaemia. In: *Irradiation as Related to Leukaemia*. National Cancer Institute Monograph **19**, 347–71.

GREITZ T., GORDON E., KOLMODIN G. & WIDEN L. (1973) Aortocranial and carotid angiography in determination of brain death. *Neuroradiology*, **5**, 13–19.

GREULICH W.W. (1960a) Value of X-ray films of hand and wrist in human identification. *Science*, **131**, 155.

GREULICH W.W. (1960b) Skeletal features visible on roentgenogram of hand and wrist which can be used for establishing individual identification. *American Journal Roentgenology*, **83**, 756.

GREULICH W.W. & PYLE S.I. (1959) *Radiographic Atlas of the Skeletal Development of the Hand and Wrist*, 2nd ed. Stanford University Press, California.

GUSTAFSON G. (1950) Age determinations on teeth. *Journal of the American Dental Association*, **41**, 45–56.

GUSTAFSON G. (1966) In: *Forensic Odontology*. Staples Press, London.

HAAS L. (1952) Roentgenological skull measurements and their diagnostic application. *American Journal Roentgenology*, **67**, 197.

HALLER J.A., JR. (1966) Injuries of the gastro-intestinal tract in children. Notes on recognition and management. *Clinical Pediatrics* (Philadelphia), **5**, 476.

HARRIS H.A. (1924) The growth of the long bones. *Proceedings of Anatomical Society*, **9**, 94.

HARRIS H.A. (1926) The growth of the long bones in childhood. *Archives of Internal Medicine*, **38**, 785–806.

HARRIS J.E., BURNOR D., LOUTFY S. & PONITZ P. (1966) A field method for the cephalometric X-ray study of skulls in early nubian cemeteries. *American Journal of Physical Anthropology*, **74**, 265–73.

HARTLEY R.C. (1967) Pancreatitis under age of five years: report of three cases. *Journal of Pediatric Surgery*, **2**, 419–23.

HARVEY W. (1946) Bite wing X-rays, a scheme for mass dental radiography. *British Journal of Radiology*, **19**, 124–6.

HARVEY W. (1975) Dental identification and forensic odontology. In: *Legal Aspects of Dental Practice* (eds. G. Forbes & A. A. Watson). John Wright & Sons Ltd., Bristol.

HARVEY W. (1976) In: *Dental Identification and Forensic Odontology*. Henry Kimpton, London.

HILL A.H. (1939) Fetal age assessment by centers of ossification. *American Journal of Physical Anthropology*, **24** (3), 251–72.

HINCK V.C. & WAGNER B.A. (1970) Informed consent. *Radiology*, **97**, 688–9.

HOLDER A.R. (1970) Law and Medicine—Angiograms. *Journal of the American Medical Association*, **213**, 349–50.

HOLDER A.R. (1972) Non-negligent failure to take X-ray films. *Journal of the American Medical Association*, **219**, 1259–60.

HOLDER A.R. (1973) Law and Medicine—Myelograms. *Journal of the American Medical Association*, **226**, 1641–2.

HUNT E.E. & GLEISER I. (1955) The estimation of age and sex of pre-adolescent children from bones and teeth. *American Journal of Physical Anthropology*, **13**, 479–487.

HUNT J.L., MCMANUS W.F., HANEY W.P. & PRUITT B.A. (1974) Vascular lesions in acute electric injuries. *The Journal of Trauma*, **14**, 461.

HUNTER T.B. & WHITEHOUSE W.M. (1974) Fresh-water near drowning: radiological aspects. *Radiology*, **112**, 51–6.

HURME V.O. (1957) Time and sequence of eruption. *Journal of Forensic Science*, **2**, 377–88.

ISRAEL H. & LEWIS A.B. (1971) Radiographically determined linear permanent tooth growth from age 6 years. *Journal of Dental Research*, **50**, 334–42.

JAMES H.E. & SCHUT L. (1974) The neurosurgeon and the battered child. *Surgical Neurology*, **2** (6), 415–8.

JENNETT B. (1976) Some medico–legal aspects of the management of acute head injury. *British Medical Journal*, **1**, 1383.

JOHANSON G. (1960) The fire catastrophe on the Haderslev estuary on July 8th 1959, and the subsequent identification. *Nordisk Kriminalteknisk. Tidskrift*, **30**, 149–56.

JOHANSON G. (1971) Age determination from human teeth. *Odontology Revue*, 22 Supplement.

JOHANSON G. & SALDEEN T. (1969) A new method for the radiological detection and identification of fragments of teeth and bone recovered from burnt victims. *Journal of Forensic Medicine*, **16**, 26–8.

KALWINSKY D., FRITELLI G. & OSKI F.A. (1974) Pancreatitis presenting as unexplained ascites. *American Journal Diseases in Childhood*, **128**, 734–6.

KEISER–NIELTEN S. (1974) New guidelines for dental recording. *International Journal of Forensic Dentistry*, **2**, 9–12.

KEMPE C.H. (1971) Paediatric implications of the battered baby syndrome. *Archives of Diseases of Childhood*, **46**, 28–37.

KEMPE C.H., SILVERMAN F.N., STEELE B.F., DROEGENMUILLER W. & SILVER H.K. (1963) Battered child syndrome. *Journal of the American Medical Association*, **181**, 17.

KING J.B. (1939) Calcification of the costal cartilages. *British Journal Radiology*, **12**, 2.

KOGON S.L. & REID J.A. (1974) The permanent identification of radiographs in forensic odontology. *Canadian Society of Forensic Science Journal*, **7**, 22–5.

KOGUTT S., SWISCHUK L.E. & FAGAN C.J. (1974) Patterns of injury and significance of uncommon fractures in the Battered Child Syndrome. *American Journal of Roentgenology*, **121** (1), 143–9.

KROGMAN W.M. (1962) *The Human Skeleton in Forensic Medicine*. Thomas Springfield, Illinois.

KROGMAN W.M. & SASSOUNI V. (1957) *A Syllabus of Roentgenographic Cephalometry*. Growth Center, University of Pennsylvania, Philadelphia.

KUNNEN, M., THOMAS, F. & VAN DE VELDE, E. (1966) Semi-microradiography of the Larynx on post-mortem material. *Medicine Science & the Law*, **6** (4), 218–9.

LACEY G., BARKER A., WIGNALL B., REIDY J. & HARPER J. (1979) Reasons for requesting radiographs in an accident department. *British Medical Journal*, **1**, 1595–7.

LACEY G. & BRADBROOKE S. (1979) Rationalising requests for X-ray examination of acute ankle injuries. *British Medical Journal*, **1**, 1597–8.

LASKER G.W. (1950) Genetic analysis of racial traits of the teeth. *Cold Spring Harbour Symposium on Quantitative Biology*, **15**, 191.

LASKER G.W. & LEE M.M.C. (1957) Racial traits in the human teeth. *Journal of Forensic Science*, **2**, 401–19.

LAW F.M. (1934) Roentgenograms as a means of identification. *American Journal Surgery*, **26**, 195.

LEEK F.F. (1971) A technique for the oral examination of a mummy. *Journal of Egyptian Archeology*, **57**, 105–9.

LEEUWEN M. VAN (1948) Post-mortem examination of teeth and supporting structures to aid in personal identification. *Archives of Pathology*, **46**, 119–27.

LOGAN W.H.G. & KRONFELD R. (1933) Development of the human jaws and surrounding structures from birth to the age of fifteen years. *Journal of the American Dental Association*, **20**, 379–427.

LOOP J.W. & BELL R.S. (1971) The utility and futility of radiographic skull examination for trauma. *New England Journal of Medicine*, **284**, 236.

LUNTZ L.L. & LUNTZ P. (1973) In: *Handbook for Dental Identification*. J. B. Lippincott Company, Philadelphia & Toronto.

MANN G.T. & FATTEH A.V. (1968) The Role of radiology in the identification of human remains: report of a case. *Journal Forensic Science Society*, **8**, 67–8.

MARESH M.M. (1940) Paranasal sinuses from birth to adolescence. *American Journal of Diseases of Children*, **60**, 55–78.

MARTEL W., WICKS J.D. & HENDRIX R.C. (1977) The accuracy of radiologic identification of humans using skeletal landmarks: a contribution to forensic pathology. *Radiology*, **124**, 681–4.

MAYER J. (1935) Identification by sinus prints. *Virginia Medical Monthly*, **62**, 517.

McCORT J. & VAUDAGNA J. (1964) Visceral injuries in battered children. *Radiology*, **82**, 424.

McKERN T.W. & STEWART T.D. (1957) Skeletal age changes in young American males, analyzed from the standpoint of identification. *Headquarters Q.M. Research and Development Command Technical Report EP–45, Natick, Massachusetts.*

THE MEDICAL DEFENCE UNION, LONDON. *Annual Reports.*

THE MEDICAL PROTECTION SOCIETY, LONDON. *Annual Reports.*

MILES A.E.W. (1958) Assessment of age from the dentition. *Proceedings of the Royal Society of Medicine*, 51, 1057–60.

MILES A.E.W. (1963) Dentition in the estimation of age. *Journal of Dental Research*, **42**, 255–63.

MILES A.E.W. (1978) Teeth as an indicator of age in man. In: *Development, Function and Evolution of Teeth* (eds. P. M. Butler and J. A. Joysey). Academic Press, London.

MILES S. (1968) Drowning. *Lancet*, **ii**, 441.

MOGG R.A. (1977) Renal artery thrombosis due to high voltage electricity. *Urologic Clinics of North America*, **4**, 13.

MOLE R.H. (1979) Radiation effects on pre-natal development and their radiological significance. *British Journal of Radiology*, **52**, 89.

MOLLISON T. (1925/6) Über die Kipfform des Mikrokephalen Mesek. *Zeitschrift für Morphologie und Anthropologie*, **24**, 109–28.

MORGAN T.A. & HARRIS M.C. (1953) Use of X-rays as an aid to medico-legal identification. *Journal Forensic Medicine*, **1**, 28.

MOORE W.J. & CORBETT M.E. (1971) The distribution of dental caries in ancient British population. *Anglo-Saxon Period Caries Research*, **5**, 151–68.

MOORREES C.F.A., FANNING E.A. & HUNT E.E. (1963) Age variation of formation stages for ten permanent teeth. *Journal of Dental Research*, **42**, 1490–502.

NAVANI S., SHAH S. & LEVY P.S. (1970) Determination of sex by costal cartilage calcification. *American Journal Roentegenology*, **108**, 771.

NEUERT W.I.A. (1931) Zu Bestimmung des Schadelinhaltes am Lebenden mit Heiffe van Rontgenbilden. *Zeitschrift für Morphogie und Anthropologie*, **20**, 261–87.

NOBACK C.R., MOSS M.L. & LESCZCYNSKA E. (1960) Digital epiphyseal fusion of the hand in adolescence: a longitudinal study. *American Journal of Physiology and Anthropology*, **18** (1), 13–18.

NOBACK C.R. & ROBERTSON G.G. (1951) Sequences of appearance of ossification centers in the human skeleton during the first five prenatal months. *American Journal of Anatomy*, **89** (1), 1–28.

NOLLA C. (1958) In: *Handbook of Orthodontics*. R. E. Moyers. Yearbook Publishers, Chicago.

OAKLEY K.P. & WEINER J.S. (1955) Piltdown Man. *American Scientist*, **43**, 573–83.

OKSANEN A. & KORMANO M. (1978) Radiology in forensic medicine: case studies. *Proceedings of the VIII International Meeting in Forensic Sciences, Wichita, Kansas.*

OSHSNER S.F. & CALONJE M.A. (1971) Reaction to intravenous iodides in nymph. *South Medical Journal,* **64,** 907–11.

PANCOAST H.K., PENDERGRASS & SCHAEFFER (1940) *The Head and Neck in Roentgen Diagnosis.* London.

PARVEY L.S. & GERALD B. (1976) Arteriographic diagnosis of brain death in children. *Pediatric Radiology,* **4,** 79–82.

PEDERSEN P.O. (1965) Forensic dentistry in Denmark. *Dental Magazine and Oral Topics,* **82,** 105–7.

PEÑA S.D.J. & MEDOVY H. (1973) Child abuse and traumatic pseudo-cyst of the pancreas. *The Journal of Pediatrics,* 1026–8.

PETERSEN K.B. & KOGAN S.L. (1971) Dental identification in the Woodbridge disaster. *Journal of the Canadian Dental Association,* **37,** 275–9.

PILLING H.H. (1976) A coroner's view of routine radiology. *Proceedings Royal Society Medicine of London,* **42,** 163.

PILLING H.H. (1976) Radiography on the investigation of death and legal proceedings. *Radiography,* **XLII,** 500, 163–6.

POOLE T.A. (1931) Reported by Mayler J. (1935) Identification by sinus prints. *Virginia Medical Monthly,* **62,** 517.

POOLE T.A. (cited by Cornwell W.S.) (1927) Radiography and photography in problems of identification: a review. *Medical Radiography and Photography,* **32** (1), 1, 34.

PUTNAM C.E., TUMMILLO A.M., MYERSON D.A. & MYERSON P.J. (1975) Drowning: another plunge. *American Journal of Roentgenology,* **125,** 543–8.

PYLE S.I. & HOERR N.L. (1955) *Radiographic Atlas of the Development of the Knee.* Thomas, Springfield, Illinois.

RAJAN R., REDDY R.D., SATHYANARAYANA K. & RAO M.D. (1976) Fracture of vertebral bodies due to accidental electric shock. *Journal Indian Medical Association,* **16,** 35.

RAVINA A.A. (1960) L'identification des corps par le V-test. *La Presse Medicale,* **68,** 178.

Recommendations of the International Commission on Radiological Protection. Annals I.C.R.P. (1977) Publication No. 26. Pergamon Press, Oxford.

RENSON C.E. (1970) The Gilstone skull. *British Dental Journal,* **128,** 95–6.

REYNOLDS E.L. (1945) The bony pelvic girdle in early infancy: a roentgenometric study. *American Journal of Physiology and Anthropology,* **3** (4), 321–54.

REYNOLDS E.L. (1947) The bony pelvis in prepubertal childhood. *American Journal of Physiology and Anthropology,* **5** (2), 165.

ROBERTS F. & SHOPFNER C.E. (1972) Plain skull roentgenograms in children with head trauma. *American Journal Roentgenology,* **114,** 230.

ROSENBAUM H.T., THOMPSON W.L. & FULLER R.H. (1964) Radiographic pulmonary changes in near-drowning. *Radiology,* **83,** 306.

ROSENKLINT A. & JØRGENSEN P.B. (1974) Evaluation of angiographic methods in the diagnosis of brain death. Correlation with local and systemic arterial pressure and intracranial pressure. *Neuroradiology*, 7, 215–9.

Royal College of Radiologists National Study (1979) Preoperative chest radiology. *Lancet*, 83–6.

RUSHTON M.A. (1965) The teeth of Anne Moubray. *British Dental Journal*, 119, 355–9.

SANDERS C.F. (1966) Sexing by costal cartilage calcification. *British Journal of Radiology*, 39, 233.

SANDERS I., WOESNER M.E., FERGUSON R.A. & NOGUCHI T.T. (1972) A new application of forensic radiology: identification of deceased from a single clavicle. *American Journal of Roentgenology*, 115, 619.

SASSOUNI V. (1955) Roentgenographic cephalometric analysis of cephalo–facio–dental relationships. *American Journal of Orthodontics*, 47, 477.

SASSOUNI V. (1957) Palatoprint, physioprint and roentgenographic cephalometry as new methods in human identification. *Journal of Forensic Science Society*, 2, 429.

SASSOUNI V. (1959) Cephalometric identification: a proposed method of identification of war dead by means of roentgenographic cephalometry. *Journal of Forensic Science Society*, 4 (1), 10.

SASSOUNI V. (1960) *The Face in Five Dimensions*. Growth Center Publications, Philadelphia.

SASSOUNI V. (1963) Dental radiography in forensic dentistry. *Journal of Dental Research*, 42, 274–302.

SAUNDERS M. (1968) Identification of the dead by the teeth. *British Dental Journal*, 124, 123–6.

SCARPELLI D.G. (1956) Fat necrosis of bone marrow in acute pancreatitis. *American Journal of Pathology*, 32, 1077.

SCHOUR I. & MASSLER M. (1941) The development of the human dentition. *Journal of the American Dental Association*, 28, 1153–60.

SCHRANZ D. (1959) Age determinations from the internal structure of the humerus. *American Journal of Physiological Anthropology* (NS), 17, 273.

SCHÜLLER A. (1921) Das Rontgengram der Stirnhole: ein Hiffsmittel für Identitätsbestimmung von Schadeln. *Monatenschrift Ohrenheilk*, 55, 1617.

SCHÜLLER A. (1943) A note on the identification of skulls by X-ray pictures of the frontal sinuses. *Medical Journal of Australia*, 1, 554–6.

SCHUSTER NORA (1968) *Manchester Medical Gazette*, 47 (3), 18–20.

SCOTT J.H. & SYMONS N.B.B. (1971) *Introduction to Dental Anatomy*. 6th ed. Churchill Livingstone, Edinburgh.

SEWARD G.R. (1972) Personal communication to Sims.

SHROFF F.R. (1959) Identification by teeth as possible source of error. *British Dental Journal*, 107, 178–80.

SHUFF R.Y. (1976) A radiographic investigation of some 19th Century skulls using a rotary cephalostat. *British Dental Journal*, 140, 343–7.

SILVERMAN F.N. (1953) The Roentgen manifestations of unrecognised skeletal trauma in infants. *American Journal of Roentgenology*, **69**, 413–26.

SIMONSEN J. (1976) Massive subarachnoid haemorrhage and fracture of the transverse process of the atlas. *Medicine Science Law*, **16**, 13–16.

SIMPSON C.K. (1978) *Police: the Investigation of Violence*—'The use of X-rays'. Macdonald and Evans, London. p. 179–97.

SINGLETON A.C. (1951) The roentgenological identification of the victims of the 'Noronic' disaster. *American Journal Roentgenology*, **66**, 375–84.

SLOVIS T., WALTER L., BERDON E., HALLER J.O., BAKER D.H. & ROSEN L. (1975) Pancreatitis and the battered child. *American Journal of Roentgenology*, **125** (2), 456–61.

SOGNNAES R.F. & STRÖM F. (1973) The odontological identification of Adolf Hitler. *Acta Odontologica Scandinavica*, **31**, 43–69.

SPARKS E.R. (1973) Reproduction of thin X-rays. *Forensic Photography*, **2**, 15–16.

SPRAWLS P. (1971) Electrocution hazards in X-ray installations. *Radiology*, **100**, 157–62.

STEVENS P.J. & TARLTON S.W. (1966) Medical investigation in fatal aircraft accidents. The role of dental evidence. *British Dental Journal*, **120**, 263–70.

STEVENSON P.H. (1924) Age order of epiphyseal union in man. *American Journal of Physiological Anthropology*, **7** (1), 53–93.

STEWART D.R., BYRD C.L. & SCHUSTER S.R. (1970) Intramural hematomas of the alimentary tract in children. *Surgery*, **68** (3), 550–7.

SWEET A.P.S. (1938) The legal aspects of dental roentgenograms. *Journal of the American Dental Association*, **25**, 1679–87.

TANNER L.E. & WRIGHT W. (1935) Recent investigations regarding the fate of the Princes in the Tower. *Archeologia*, **84**, 1–26.

TCHAPEROFF I.C.C. (1937) *A Manual of Radiological Diagnosis for Students and General Practitioners*. Wood, Baltimore.

THOMAS H. & GREULICH W.W. (1940) A comparative study of male and female pelves. *American Journal of Obstetrics and Gynecology*, **39**, 56–62.

THOMSON J.L.G. (1955) Enlargement of the Sella Turcica: Report on 27 cases. *British Journal of Radiology*, **28**, 454–61.

THORNE H.H. & THYBERG H. (1953) Identification of children or adults by means of mass minature radiography of the cranium. *Acta Odontologica Scandanavica*, **11** (2), 129.

TODD T.W. (1920) Age changes in the pubic bone. 1: the male white pubis. *American Journal of Physical Anthropology*, **3** (3), 285–334.

TODD T.W. (1921) Age changes in the pubic bone: II the pubis of the male Negro-white hybrid. III the pubis of the white female. IV the pubis of the female Negro-white hybrid. *American Journal of Physical Anthropology*, **4** (1), 1–70.

TODD T.W. (1921) Age changes in the pubic bone: V Mammalian pubic metamorphosis. *American Journal of Physical Anthropology*, **4** (4), 333–406.

TODD T.W. (1921) Age changes in the pubic bone: VI the interpretation of variations in the symphysial area. *American Journal of Physical Anthropology*, **4** (4), 407–24.

TODD T.W. (1923) Age changes in the pubic symphysis: VII The anthropoid strain in human pubic symphyses of the third decade. *American Journal of Physical Anthropology*, **57** (3), 274–94.

TODD T.W. (1930) Age changes in the pubic bone: VIII Roentgeno-graphic differentiation. *American Journal of Physical Anthropology*, **14** (2), 255–71.

TOULOUKIAN T.J. (1968) Abdominal visceral injuries in battered children. *Pediatrics*, **42** (4), 642–6.

TRATMAN E.K. (1938) Three rooted lower molars in man and their racial distribution. *British Dental Journal*, **64**, 264–74.

TURPIN R., TISSERAND M. (1942) Etude correlative des sinus. Fron-taux des Jumeaux. *Compte Rendu de la Société Biologie*, **136**, 203.

ULIN A.W., OLSEN A.K. & MARTIN W.L. (1955) Factors determining mortality in patients with acute head injury. *The Journal of the American Medical Association*, **157**, 496.

VANEZIS P. (1979) Techniques used in the evaluation of vertebral trauma at post-mortem. *Forensic Science International*, **13**, 159–65.

VOIGT G.E. (1961) Fatal basal subarachnoid haemorrhage following an occupational accident. *Monatsschrift Unfallheilkunde*, **64**, 21–23.

VOLUTER G. (1959) The 'V' test. *Radiologica Clinica*, Basel. **28**, 1–32.

VOLUTER (cited by Ravina, A.) (1960) L'identification des corps par le V-test. *Le Presse Medicale*, **68**, 178.

WAALER E. (1960) Identifisering au dödsofrere ether brannen pa Stalheim Turisthotell i junr 1959. *Norske Tannlaegepren Tidscrift*, **70**, 513–26.

WATSON A.A. (1974) Estimation of age from skeletal remains. *Journal of the Forensic Science Society*, **14**, 209–13.

WESENBERG R.L., GWINN J.L., BARNES G.R. JR. (1969) Radiological findings in the kinky-hair syndrome. *Radiology*, **92**, 500–6.

WHITTAKER D.K. (1977) Identification by means of teeth. *British Journal of Surgical Technicians*, **1**, 45–51.

WHITTAKER D.K. (1980) The use of tooth fragments in species deter-mination. *British Dental Journal*, **148**, 105–6.

WHITTAKER D.K., ROTHWELL T., SAMBROOK S.C., STUCKEY I.C. & TREHARNE D. (1978) Species determination from tooth frag-ments. *British Dental Journal*, **144**, 81–2.

WOOLLEY P.V. & EVANS W.A. (1955) Significance of skeletal lesions in infants resembling those of traumatic origin. *Journal of the Ameri-can Medical Association*, **158**, 539–43.

WORTH H.M. (1963) *Principles and Practice of Oral Radiologic Interpre-tation.* Year Book Medical Publishers Incorporated.

WULLENWEBER R., SCHNEIDER W. & GRUMME T. (1977) Computerised tomography in the study of intracranial bullet lesions (Germ). *Zeitschrift Rechtsmedizin*, **80**, 227.

YAMAMOTO K., KARJIURA K. & TOKI S. (1971) Differentiation between human and animal teeth by means of scanning electron micro-scopy. *Bulletin of the Tokyo Dental College*, **12**, 317–32.

Young L.W. & Adams J.T. (1967) Roentgenographic findings in localised trauma to pancreas in children. *American Journal of Roentgenology. RAD Therapy & Nuclear Medicines,* **101**, 639–48.

Index

Note: Figures in **bold** type refer to pages on which illustrations appear.

DATE DUE

APR 1 9 '05		
OCT 2 3 2007		
NOV 1 4 2007		
FEB 1 4 2008		

GAYLORD   #3522PI   Printed in USA